Nuclear Medicine:
Self Study Program II
INSTRUMENTATION

Series Editors

Peter T. Kirchner, MD
University of Iowa Hospitals and Clinics

Barry A. Siegel, MD
Mallinckrodt Institute of Radiology

Self-Study Program II
Editor

L. Stephen Graham, PhD
West Los Angeles VA Medical Center

Contributors

Anthony R. Benedetto, PhD
University of Kentucky Medical Center

Gerd Muehllehner, PhD
UGM Medical Systems

David R. Pickens, PhD
Vanderbilt University Medical Center

NUCLEAR MEDICINE: SELF-STUDY PROGRAM II

INSTRUMENTATION

- Syllabus
- References
- Multiple-Choice Questions
- Answers and Critiques for Multiple-Choice Questions

Society of Nuclear Medicine
1850 Samuel Morse Drive, Reston, Virginia 20190-5316

Made in the United States of America.

Library of Congress Cataloging in Publication Data

Kirchner, Peter T.
Nuclear medicine: self-study program II: instrumentation/Peter T. Kirchner, Barry A. Siegel
Includes bibliographical references and index
ISBN 0-932004-44-X (pbk.)
1. Nuclear medicine—Instruments—Programmed instruction.
I. Siegel, Barry, 1944- . II. Title.
[DNLM: 1. Nuclear Medicine—instrumentation. 2. Diagnostic Imaging—Instrumentation. 3. Technology, Radiologic—instrumentation WN 440 K575n 1996]
R920.K57 1996
616.07'575—dc20
DNLM/DLC
for Library of Congress **95-48204**
CIP

Contents

Instrumentation

INTRODUCTION

Significant changes in the appearance and performance of nuclear medicine instrumentation have occurred over the past 10 years. These changes have come about as a result of the incorporation of integrated circuits and the appropriate software as well as other technical advances. The improved performance of these instruments has expanded their utilization in all aspects of nuclear medicine, but their increased complexity makes it timely to review both their enhanced capabilities and limitations.

This syllabus briefly reviews the basic principles of operation of state-of-the-art nonimaging and imaging instruments and computers and provides information on performance parameters as they directly relate to clinical usage.

NONIMAGING INSTRUMENTATION

Radiation Protection Instruments

In nuclear medicine, radiation protection instruments are used either to detect the presence of radioactive contamination or to quantify the radiation emitted by radiopharmaceuticals located in storage areas, in radioactive waste, or in patients. In general, Geiger-Muller (G-M) detectors are better suited for the detection of small amounts of radioactivity, whereas ionization chambers are better suited for measuring high radiation levels and accurately measuring exposure rates (milliroentgens per hour [mR/hr]).

Geiger-Muller Detectors. Geiger-Muller detectors are gas-filled detectors that operate at high voltages (750–1100 V); the large amplitude of the output pulse of a G-M detector is due to the millionfold multiplication of the ionization signal that occurs when the gas detector completely discharges. This complete discharge leads to a readily detectable output signal, but it also contributes to the relatively long dead time (the time during which another event cannot be processed) of a G-M detector. From a practical standpoint, a G-M detector has such a long dead time that it can be used reliably only when the number of beta particles or gamma rays striking it is relatively small. If the radiation field is too intense, the observed count rate may be substantially lower than the actual number of interactions within the detector.

Several types of G-M tubes can be purchased with an instrument. End-window tubes have thin mica entrance windows that permit the passage of relatively low energy ("soft") particles into the chamber. Many tubes of this type have removable covers so that penetrating radiations can be separated from nonpenetrating radiations. Other tubes are designed for counting relatively penetrating radiations and have thicker, more sturdy walls. Pancake probes are designed for monitoring equipment and laboratory surfaces and have a large (approximately 20 cm^2) surface area.

Laboratory monitors and most G-M survey meters use large G-M detectors to maximize sensitivity, to enhance their ability to detect small amounts of contamination on hands, clothes and work areas. Their use should be restricted to the detection of contamination. They should never be used when accurate quantitation of exposure rates is necessary.

Licensees who use technetium generators or who routinely have very large quantities of radiopharmaceuticals on hand, especially for radionuclide therapy, are required to have at least one instrument capable of measuring up to 1,000 mR/hr. Special G-M survey meters are available with this operating range.

Ionization Chamber Detectors. The long dead time and energy dependence of G-M detectors renders them unsuitable for accurate measurement of radiation levels, especially at high exposure rates (above 100 mR/hr). Accuracy is the province of ionization chamber instruments.

Ionization chamber survey meters also use gas-filled detectors. The gas is usually ordinary room air at ambient temperature and pressure. If ionizing events occur continuously and in large numbers, the total charge of all the electrons collected will be sufficiently large to generate a current, albeit a very small one (on the order of 10^{-12} A [1 pA]). Sensitive current-measuring devices called electrometers are used to accurately measure these small currents. The corresponding exposure rate or integrated exposure value is displayed digitally or on an analog meter. Even ionization chambers show some energy dependence. An energy response curve that relates photon energy to indicated versus actual exposure rate is normally provided with each instrument.

One type of ionization chamber survey meter is identified by the name "Cutie Pie." It has a small-diameter (approximately 7 cm), long (30–40 cm) cylindrical chamber with a pistol-grip handle that contains the electronic circuits, a meter, and the controls. Recently, an air ion chamber in a different configuration has become available that utilizes CMOS thyroid microprocessor technology and a liquid-crystal display. It is much more compact and lighter in weight than the Cutie Pie. Ionization chamber survey meters are more expensive than G-M survey meters but are the instrument of choice for measuring exposure rates in unrestricted areas, determining the labeling requirements for shipments of packages containing radioactive materials, and estimating the radioiodine burden of a patient with carcinoma to decide when he or she can legally and safely be discharged from the hospital.

Pocket ionization chambers are sometimes used to measure integrated exposure for personnel who care for patients undergoing radiation therapy. Because of their small size (approximately 1.5 cm in diameter, 10 cm long), these devices can be clipped to a shirt pocket or collar and be read by the user, thus providing an immediate indication of exposure. Pocket ionization chambers are susceptible to mechanical shock and only read exposures down to 10 mR with an accuracy of about 20%.

Radionuclide Calibrators

When radioactivity levels of 50 kBq (roughly 1 μCi) or less must be measured accurately, the sodium iodide [NaI(Tl)] detector should be used (see Sodium Iodide-Based Systems). At higher activities, however, NaI(Tl) detectors exhibit severe dead-time losses and can be used only by making large dead-time corrections of dubious accuracy. Large activities, in the kilobecquerel to gigabecquerel (microcurie to curie) range, must be measured with a radionuclide calibrator, usually referred to as a dose calibrator.

All commercial radionuclide calibrators contain a reentrant-well ionization chamber filled with either room air at ambient pressure or argon at a pressure of 12 atm. The ambient air design can measure large activities. The pressurized chamber is more sensitive and thus better suited for measuring low activities; it also has less dependence on geometry (i.e., there is less variability when a given activity is measured in a large vial or small syringe). Activities below 15–25 μCi (0.5–1 MBq) are not accurately assayed in a radionuclide calibrator and should be measured by dilution using a NaI(Tl) detector.

In an analog radionuclide calibrator, the conversion from current to activity is accomplished by proper selection of a resistance through which the ionization chamber current flows, so that the reading on the display is calibrated in activity units (curies, becquerels). In commercial radionuclide calibrators, a digital 10-turn potentiometer, which is simply a high-accuracy variable resistor, allows any value of resistance to be selected by the operator according to a conversion table provided by the manufacturer. Push-button switches are provided for the instant selection of the more common radionuclides; the buttons insert a resistor of the required value into the current-to-activity conversion circuit.

Digital radionuclide calibrators digitize the ionization chamber current with an analog-to-digital converter (ADC). The operator conveys radionuclide identity to a microprocessor through a menu or with a coded key. The manufacturer will have provided the current-to-activity conversion factor for each radionuclide in a lookup table in either a floppy disk data file or in a customized read-only memory (ROM) chip. The microprocessor retrieves the appropriate conversion factor, multiplies it by the current, and displays the activity on a video monitor.

Separate desktop microcomputers or onboard microprocessors can be used with both analog and digital radionuclide calibrators to perform a number of calculational and recordkeeping functions. For example, the volume and activity of the generator eluate could be entered immediately after elution. If the time of the activity measurement is maintained by an internal clock, the computer can generate a database file that can be queried at any time during the day at for the current activity.

As aliquots are drawn for the reconstitution of kits (e.g., methylene diphosphonate [MDP], sulfur colloid) or for patient dosages, the computer can make a record of each withdrawal and can update the generator eluate database file with new volume data. Then, if the operator wishes to withdraw a given dosage later in the day, the computer would calculate the decay factor and the volume to be withdrawn. It appears that such computer records will be acceptable to regulatory agencies, but great care will need to be taken to ensure that floppy disk, tape, or optical disk backup copies are maintained continuously in case of floppy or hard disk failure.

A radionuclide calibrator will report an activity reading for any source of radioactivity whose radiations penetrate the counting gas and interact to produce ion pairs. If the calibrator has been set to measure the activity of thallium-201, but a vial of gallium-67 is placed in the chamber, the calibrator will faithfully measure the current, multiply it by the conversion factor for thallium-201, and display an incorrect activity reading. Radionuclide calibrators contain no pulse height analysis capability. An alert technologist should detect the discrepancy between the activity given by the vendor (or calculated for a kit) and the activity shown by the calibrator. There are no comforting multichannel analyzer displays or windows, such as are found in most gamma cameras and NaI(Tl) well counters.

Because it lacks a pulse height analyzer, a radionuclide calibrator does not have the ability to electronically reject stray radiation. This sensitivity to stray radiation is aggravated by the fact that most calibrators are located in the nuclear pharmacy, close to generators, stock vials, waste, and dosage preparation areas. The first line of defense is to purchase the customized lead shield that is available as an accessory for every calibrator; this shield also provides extra protection for nuclear pharmacy workers. If an instrument is purchased without the shield, addition of a shield requires that the dose calibrator be recalibrated. Failure to do so will produce inaccurate, falsely high readings. The second line of defense is placement of the calibrator as far from radioactivity use and storage areas as possible. Patients can be potent sources of stray radiation, so the calibrator should not be too close to imaging, waiting, or rest rooms or hallways frequented by patients. The third line of defense is the technologist, who should always ensure that the display of the calibrator reads essentially zero before each measurement.

The technologist should not indiscriminately use the *background* control because the stray radiation may be due to contamination of the reentrant well's plastic liner. Contamination should be suspected if the calibrator did not exhibit high background radiation levels during the early morning quality control testing. Most well liners are easy to remove and decontaminate.

The response of a radionuclide calibrator can vary significantly, depending on the geometry of the radioactive material placed in its reentrant well. For example, a full 1-ml syringe containing 100 mCi of technetium-99m will give a substantially different activity reading than 100 mCi of technetium-99m in a full 60-ml syringe. Fortunately, most nuclear medicine dosages are drawn into 1-, 3-, or 5-ml syringes, and there are only small differences (5% or less) in readings for these three syringes when each contains a dose of 100 mCi. There can be substantial differences in calibrator readings of identical doses placed in plastic syringes and glass stock vials, especially for radionuclides whose photons have energies below 100 keV and for beta-emitting radionuclides. All expected source geometries must be tested during acceptance testing, and any correction factors greater than 10% must be posted on or near the calibrator and used in clinical practice.

Some vendors of radionuclide calibrators may represent their instruments as capable of measuring the activity of phosphorus-32, which emits only beta particles. Bremsstrahlung production in glass is not an efficient process, but clinical dosages of phosphorus-32 usually involve millicurie quantities, and the total number of beta particles interacting in the glass is high. The bremsstrahlung photons can have energies up to 1,700 keV, with most occurring around 500 keV, and these photons can easily enter the ionization chamber and interact in the counting gas. Correction factors for phosphorus-32 will be strongly dependent on the source geometry, so that a 1-ml plastic syringe containing 1 ml will give a vastly different reading than that same 1 ml of solution in its glass stock vial. Measurement of phosphorus-32 activity can be accomplished with a radionuclide calibrator, but its use requires meticulous attention to source geometry.

Quality Control Testing. The radionuclide calibrator is the primary instrument for verifying that the radiopharmaceutical dosage prepared for administration to the patient is the actual dosage prescribed by the nuclear physician. Proper operation of the radionuclide calibrator must be ensured by the performance of routine testing of constancy, linearity, and accuracy. Results of quality control testing must be reviewed promptly to determine whether an equipment malfunction has occurred.

Constancy. On completion of acceptance testing of a new radionuclide calibrator, a long-lived solid-sealed source (usually cobalt-57 or cesium-137) is designated as a constancy check source for the purpose of verifying day-to-day stability of the instrument. The source is placed in the calibrator, and its "activity" is measured using the common radionuclide buttons and potentiometer settings. Each day, before use of the calibrator for patient dosages, the constancy check source is assayed on all commonly used settings, and the readings are recorded and compared with the decay-corrected benchmark values.

Linearity. Radionuclide calibrators should display the correct activity throughout the full range of activities used in the nuclear medicine clinic (e.g., a generator eluate of 70 GBq, a patient dosage of 40 MBq, or a gamma-camera intrinsic flood source of 4 MBq). Two different methods are accepted by regulatory agencies for performing a linearity test. One requires periodic assays of a decaying source of technetium-99m over a period of 3 to 5 days. The other involves simulating the decay of technetium-99m by the use of a series of calibrated lead sleeves that are placed over the source. The disadvantage of the former is the time required to complete the test. The latter can be completed in 5 to 10 min, but the results may be different when high activity levels are used than when the test is performed with low activity levels. All regulatory agencies require that the linearity test be performed at installation and every 3 months thereafter. Specific instructions for performing these tests and the methods of analysis are described in regulatory guides published by the Nuclear Regulatory Commission (NRC) or the state licensing agency.

Accuracy. Accuracy can be defined as the agreement between the radionuclide calibrator reading and the known activity of a radionuclide in a standard vial or syringe configuration. The data are acquired by making three independent measurements of each source and calculating the average value. A full accuracy test must be performed at least annually. The test must be repeated after any major repair of the dose calibrator.

The calibrator should be tested with two or three radionuclides, and at least two sources should have different principal photon energies (e.g., cobalt-57, cesium-137, or cobalt-60). At least one of the radionuclides must have a principal photon energy between 100 and 500 keV. These sources must have an activity level of at least 50 μCi. Ideally, these sources should be purchased directly from the National Institute of Standards and Technology (NIST, formerly the National Bureau of Standards); if NIST sources are not available, the sources from another supplier should be furnished with a calibration certificate showing traceability to NIST. The calibrator reading must be ±5% of the source activity. Cobalt-57 and barium-133 sources will occasionally give readings slightly above +5% due to the high abundance of soft x-rays that penetrate the plastic vials.

Sodium Iodide–Based Systems

The nonimaging sodium iodide–based systems normally found in nuclear medicine clinics include well counters, uptake probes, and various types of regional counters. Each system may contain 1–24 thallium-doped sodium iodide NaI(Tl) crystals (each with its own photomultiplier tube [PMT], high-voltage supply, preamplifier, and amplifier), one or more single-channel or multichannel pulse height analyzers, lead shielding or collimation to reduce stray and background radiation, and, more and more, a desktop or integral microcomputer to acquire and analyze the counting data obtained.

Single Sample Well Counters. Single sample well counters are used for counting a wide variety of samples, ranging from iodine-125-labeled human serum albumin (35 keV; plasma volume) to cobalt-57 (122 keV; Schilling test) to iodine-131 (364 keV; effective renal plasma flow) to iron-59 (1,300 keV; ferrokinetics).

For a small sample located at the bottom of the well, the counting geometry is almost 4π, and the counting efficiency is maximized. The metal protective casing around the crystal prevents the entrance of light and moisture. It is made of aluminum, a low-Z material that allows low-energy photons to penetrate the crystal, where they are efficiently absorbed. Efficiency for counting high-energy gamma rays is maximized by making the outer diameter of the NaI(Tl) crystal large (up to 7.5 cm) and the diameter of the well small, thus providing a large path length for photon absorption in the NaI(Tl) crystal. The NaI(Tl) crystal and the PMT are usually supplied as a single integrated unit. The preamplifier is frequently contained within the base into which the PMT pins are plugged. The crystal-PMT-preamplifier assembly is enclosed in a massive lead shield to protect against natural background radiation and stray radiation from radioactive material in the vicinity of the detector system.

The simplest, least expensive pulse height analysis device is a single-channel analyzer (SCA). The operator sets a lower level energy discriminator and an upper level energy discriminator, or a window, so that only photons whose energies fall within the desired energy range are recorded.

A more expensive pulse height analyzer is the multichannel analyzer (MCA). In an MCA the detector output pulse is digitized and parsed into an appropriate memory cell based on the photon energy absorbed in the crystal; the resulting spectrum is displayed in real time on a cathode ray tube (CRT). The operator uses an electronic cursor to define any desired number of energy windows, using the peaks of the spectrum and the calibrated energy scale of the MCA as guides in selecting the correct peaks and proper window width. The MCA automatically sums all the counts within the window and displays them on the CRT. Because they may have from 100 to more than 8,000 individual channels, MCAs are usually interfaced to printers or computers; manual recording would be extremely tedious and fraught with transcription errors.

The analysis of NaI(Tl) well counter data may be manual or automated by use of an accessory computer into which data must be entered manually, by use of an accessory computer that receives data through a hard-wired connection from the pulse height analyzer, or by a computer in which the MCA is installed in an expansion slot. Multichannel analyzers are now available on a single printed circuit board such that the MCA board is controlled by its own dedicated onboard microprocessor and runs completely independently of the desktop microcomputer in which it is installed. Data storage is accomplished on the host computer's disks (floppy or hard), and data are very rapidly uploaded into the host computer's memory for processing.

The accuracy of data obtained from a well counter is limited by two factors: sample volume and count rate. A large volume of material containing a uniformly distributed radionuclide will produce a lower count rate than a small volume. This lower count rate is due to self-absorption and a difference in geometry relative to the detector material. At high count rates, coincidence losses become significant because of the simultaneous arrival of two or more photons. Because all photons that interact with the crystal must be processed, reducing the size of the pulse height analyzer window does not eliminate the losses.

Thyroid Uptake Probes. A basic thyroid uptake probe system consists of a flat-faced NaI(Tl) crystal with a single PMT and preamplifier, a high-voltage power supply, an amplifier, a SCA, a scaler, a lead shield around the back and sides of the detector assembly, and an open-field collimator facing the patient. Modern thyroid uptake systems are optimized for iodine-123 (159-keV gamma rays) rather than iodine-131 (364-keV gamma rays), and data analysis is much more highly automated. The NaI(Tl) crystals are 5–7.5 cm in diameter and 5 cm thick because of the lower penetrating power of iodine-123 gamma rays. Stand-alone "smart" MCAs or conventional MCAs coupled to microcomputers are the standard methods of pulse height analysis. Smart MCAs have limited computational power and built-in firmware to calculate thyroid uptake and other typical radioassay applications involving sample counting (e.g., Schilling test).

Thyroid counting requires meticulous attention to the accurate positioning of the detector in relation to both the neck phantom and the patient's neck (20–30 cm). Some collimators are long enough that the proper geometry is achieved by simply placing the end of the collimator against the phantom or the patient's neck and thigh. The collimator opening is usually wide enough to allow visual verification that the thyroid is completely within its field of view. Proper positioning can be ensured by repositioning the collimator until the maximum count rate is achieved. If the collimator is shorter than the required separation distance (20–30 cm), a means must be provided to indicate the necessary distance from the face of the collimator to the skin surface.

If thyroid uptake studies are peformed in patients who have received scan doses of iodine-123 (as much as 400 μCi of iodine-123), coincidence losses may produce falsely low uptake values. A set of correction factors can be produced by placing the maximum activity of iodine-123 in a thyroid phantom and monitoring the observed count rate as a function of time. By plotting the observed count rate versus time on semilogarithmic paper and extrapolating the straight-line portion of the data at low activity levels to the maximum activity, correction factors can be obtained.

Multisample Gamma Counters. The earliest multisample gamma counters used NaI(Tl) well counters and simply added conveyor belts, sample elevators, and hard-copy printout devices. An important advantage of these systems, with their large NaI(Tl) detectors and massive lead shielding, was their ability to count the relatively high-energy gamma rays from iodine-131, iron-59, cobalt-58, cobalt-57, and technetium-99m, as well as the low-energy x-rays and gamma rays from iodine-125.

Over the years, two distinct classes of multisample gamma counters have emerged. One class still utilizes a large crystal and massive shielding and is found predominantly in research institutions and in laboratories where radionuclides that emit high-energy photons are used. The other class is tailored for iodine-125. These machines can count cobalt-57 and technetium-99m but with substantial loss of counting efficiency and overall machine throughput. These machines designed for iodine-125 typically have multiple NaI(Tl) well detectors (up to 24), each only a few centimeters in diameter and with only minimal lead shielding between detectors.

All modern multisample gamma counters are designed to be microprocessor controlled throughout all stages of operation, from sample movement and selection through recording and processing of counting data. Some systems can count radioimmunoassay standards, derive, and plot the standard curve; perform and record quality control calculations; calculate actual sample concentrations; and print out group and individual patient reports.

Quality Control Testing. The NaI(Tl) detector systems described in this section have well-defined and circumscribed roles in a nuclear medicine clinic. The number of different radionuclides counted is generally small, and the sample geometries are fairly standard. These characteristics allow a quality control testing program to be simpler and less involved than might be the case for similar instruments in the health physics laboratory of a large research institution.

Peaking (Daily). Peaking is the verification that the energy window is positioned properly on the photopeak. For an SCA, the clinically used radionuclide (in a scatter-free geometry) is placed in or on the detector, the energy window is set, and the amplifier fine gain or high voltage is adjusted until the count rate is maximal (i.e., the photopeak is properly positioned). This task is easier in an MCA, because the operator can visually monitor a shift of the photopeak into the window to correct for slight changes in the kiloelectron volt/channel calibration.

Constancy (Daily). This check is very similar in concept to the daily radionuclide calibrator constancy check. A long-lived source, whose actual activity need not be accurately known, is counted at the time of the annual energy calibration, and a counts-per-minute per becquerel (microcurie) factor is determined. Thereafter, this source is counted daily before clinical use, and the counts-per-minute per becquerel (microcurie) value is calculated and compared with the "true" value. A change of 10% or more in this value would indicate a change in gain or high voltage or could indicate a damaged detector or malfunctioning electronics, and repair should be made promptly.

Reproducibility or Precision (Monthly). If a long-lived source is counted repeatedly by a properly functioning detector, the resulting individual counts will not be identical; rather, they will be grouped about a mean value according to a Poisson distribution. Thus, one of the checks for proper operation of a detector is to determine whether repeated counts of a source yield a Poisson distribution. The preferred test is the chi-square test, which uses a Gaussian distribution as an approximation of a Poisson distribution.

When the data are analyzed, two types of failures may be encountered. A low p value (<0.05) indicates that there is only a small probability that a Poisson distribution would give the same chi-square value as large as was observed. The large value may be produced by electronic noise. A high p value (>0.95) is also undesirable because it indicates that random variations are much smaller than those of a Poisson distribution. If either of these results are obtained, the first step is to repeat the test. If similar values are obtained, service should be requested.

Energy calibration (semiannual). For instruments that count radionuclides other than iodine-125, it is convenient to calibrate the gain setting of the amplifier or the high voltage so that the SCA/MCA energy window dial settings or the electronic cursor are calibrated to a convenient kiloelectron-volt per channel setting. In SCAs with 10-turn potentiometers, the usual energy range is 0–1,000 keV, so that the dial settings read directly in kiloelectron volts. Most MCAs in nuclear medicine have 1024, 2048, or 4096 channels, with 1024 channels and 1 keV per channel being a common combination.

Energy calibration for an SCA entails placing a gamma-ray source (usually cesium-137) in the detector, setting the energy window to a very narrow setting (typically ±5 to ±10 keV around the photopeak energy), and using the amplifier fine-gain or high-voltage setting to move the gamma-ray photopeak up or down along the energy scale until the measured photopeak is perfectly centered in the narrow window. The gain and high-voltage settings are noted on a worksheet or in a logbook. Energy calibration for an MCA is less tedious. Because the spectrum is shown in real time during acquisition, and the cursor can be placed exactly on the channel corresponding to the photopeak energy, sliding the peak into the desired channel is easily done.

It should be kept in mind that NaI(Tl) detector systems may not be linear over the range 0–1,000 keV. For example, if the 662-keV gamma ray of cesium-

137 appears in channel 662, the 122-keV gamma ray from cobalt-57 may be in channel 124 or 125. Wide windows are used in nuclear medicine, and the energy resolution of NaI(Tl) is not very good, so a shift of a few kiloelectron volts is not detrimental for clinical applications.

Energy resolution (annual). Because of the hygroscopic nature of NaI(Tl) crystals, energy resolution should be checked on a regular basis. The presence of moisture in the crystal causes it to turn yellow, which interferes with the transmission of light from the crystal to the PMT. Although different radionuclides can be used, this test is usually performed with cesium-137. Data consist of a series of measurements made with a narrow pulse height analyzer window (typically 20 keV) from a point where the counts are less than 50% of the maximum on the low side of the energy range to where they are less than 50% of the maximum on the high side. The position of the window for individual measurements should be such that it does not overlap other measurements and that there are no gaps in the energy range covered. The full width at half maximum (FWHM) of this data set should be less than 10% for cesium-137.

Efficiency or sensitivity (annual). The terms "efficiency" and "sensitivity" are used synonymously herein. The purpose of determining a detector's efficiency is to allow the conversion of observed photopeak counts to activity (in becquerels or microcuries). The efficiency of a sodium iodide detector can be expressed in two slightly different ways:

1. A sample with NIST-traceable activity is counted using the energy window setting to be used clinically. The conversion factor from count rate to activity is calculated by dividing the observed net count rate (counts per minute) by the known activity of the sample (becquerels or microcuries). This efficiency calibration method requires the use of actual clinically used radionuclides, some of which may be difficult and expensive to acquire with NIST-traceable calibration.
2. A more general efficiency calibration results in a curve of observed counts per incident gamma ray as a function of gamma-ray energy. Typically, plastic rods that approximate test tube geometry and that contain NIST-traceable activities in a point source configuration are used. Sets of these rod sources are available with energies ranging from 30 keV (iodine-129) to 1.33 MeV (cobalt-60). The efficiency factor for a given gamma-ray energy is then the observed net count rate (counts per minute) divided by the gamma-ray emission rate (gamma rays per minute). Because the rod source sets typically do not contain the clinically important radionuclides, the efficiency factors for the various energies are plotted as a function of energy in the form of a smooth "efficiency" curve, and the efficiency for the clinically used gamma-ray energy is read from the curve by interpolation.

Xenon Respirometer/Trap

Radionuclides of xenon gas (xenon-133 and xenon-127) are used for assessment of pulmonary ventilation. A dosage of 10–20 rCi (40–70 MBq) is administered during a single deep inhalation. The patient exhales the xenon into a respirometer and rebreathes the xenon/air mixture for about 5 min. At the end of the rebreathing period, the patient exhales the xenon/air mixture and inhales room air. The exhaled xenon is either dispersed by dilution to the environment or by delay and decay in a xenon "trap."

A xenon trap is composed of canisters filled with activated charcoal through which the exhaled xenon/air mixture is pulled by a small pump. Xenon is an inert gas and undergoes adsorption–desorption as it slowly moves through the charcoal. The charcoal mass, temperature, total integrated volume of air pulled through the trap by the pump, and total linear distance the xenon must traverse through the charcoal determine the time required for the xenon to travel from the intake of the trap to the outlet. Commercial traps are designed to allow for substantial decay of 5-day half-life xenon-133 before it works its way to the outlet. The pump should be run only during collection of a patient's exhaled xenon because its operation at other times serves to hasten the movement of xenon through the trap.

As a general rule of thumb, when the effluent from a trap exceeds 1 mR/hr, or it has been used for 2 years, the charcoal canister should be replaced. Even though the bound radioactivity will finally decay to background levels, the charcoal should not be reused because many of the sites are occupied by moisture and airborne contaminants and are no longer available for binding xenon. Used canisters must be stored in a shielded area and sealed in plastic bags before final disposal.

The longer half-life and higher energy photons of xenon-127 (36 days, 172,203 keV) will not be adequately addressed in xenon traps designed for xenon-133. The use of xenon-127 dictates additional lead shielding and more canisters (because of the longer decay time required) and thus more frequent canister changes. Regardless of the radionuclide used, the trap should be equipped with a radiation detector to alert the operator that excessive amounts of radioactive xenon are being released.

Liquid Scintillation Counter

Biomedical research relies heavily on hydrogen-3 (tritium) and carbon-14 because of their long half-lives and the relative ease with which they can be used as radiolabels of biologically important molecules. The quantitation of tritium and carbon-14 is hampered by the very weak beta particles that are emitted. The most efficient way to count tritium and carbon-14 (and most other beta-emitting radionuclides) is to dissolve or disperse the biological specimen in a solution that scintillates when it absorbs the beta particles. With the proper scintillation fluid, the light emitted is proportional to beta-particle energy, and beta spectrometry can be performed. In a liquid scintillation counter, a vial containing the sample and scintillation fluid (sometimes called a cocktail) is lowered into a light-tight compartment shielded from background and stray radiation by several centimeters of lead. The vial is viewed by two PMTs operated in coincidence to reduce noise from PMT dark current and from nonsample radiation striking the photoemissive surfaces within the PMT. The PMT output pulse is subjected to pulse height analysis by either one to three SCAs or one MCA. Modern liquid scintillation counters have onboard microprocessors to control data acquisition and processing; the most advanced models are multiuser and multitasking and operate with very little human intervention.

The process of transforming beta-particle kinetic energy into the light that strikes the PMT photocathode is multistep and is sensitive to many factors. Chemical contaminants, undesired colorants, and sample self-absorption are examples of factors that reduce the amount of light reaching the PMT (*quenching*). Quenching causes the pulse height analyzer to think that it is receiving lower energy beta-particle energies, thereby negatively affecting its ability to perform spectrometry. Liquid scintillation counters are equipped with proprietary methods for correcting for quenching effects. The use of these correction techniques is mandatory for accurate and reproducible results.

Liquid scintillation cocktails originally were based on toluene, benzene, naphthalene, and other toxic organic chemicals. Newly introduced cocktails are water soluble and do not contain high levels of these objectionable chemicals. These new cocktails can be disposed of in the sanitary sewage system if the activity concentration is below specified levels.

Regional Cerebral Blood Flow Probe Systems

Regional cerebral metabolism can be assessed only by positron emission tomography (PET); single-photon methods simply do not exist at this time. Changes in regional cerebral blood flow (rCBF) are correlated with changes in regional cerebral metabolism in normal subjects and in most patients with clinically important illnesses. Imaging and nonimaging methods of estimating rCBF using xenon-133, iodine-123–labeled iodoamphetamine (IMP), and technetium-99m–labeled hexamethylpropyleneamine oxime (HMPAO), are available.

When radioactive xenon is introduced into the cerebral circulation by injection or inhalation, it is removed from the bloodstream by the gray and white matter. The rates of inflow and outflow in gray matter are faster than the rates in white matter by roughly a factor of 4. A radiation detector viewing a defined region of the brain generates an activity–time curve of the inflow and outflow of the radioactive xenon from which gray and white matter flow rates can be calculated.

Whole-brain or hemispheric rCBF can be measured by placing the patient's head into a "helmet" to which are affixed up to 32 small collimated NaI(Tl) detectors. A dedicated computer controls the administration of xenon, acquisition of the probe data and other data needed for analysis, and deconvolution of the activity–time curves to derive gray and white matter flow rates. The process is fully automated and results in a map of rCBF in each type of brain tissue.

The measurement of rCBF by this method is relatively straightforward and of adequate precision to permit observation of small changes after intervention or during the course of long-term illness. The major disadvantages are the lack of an image, poor spatial resolution because of detector size and detector field-of-view limitations, and the use of a radioactive gas. Only imaging techniques are used to evaluate rCBF with iodine-123–labeled IMP and technetium-99m–labeled HMPAO.

ANGER SCINTILLATION CAMERAS

Introduction

Anger scintillation cameras have become the major imaging instrument in nuclear medicine, due to, in part, the high spatial resolution and contrast that these instruments can now provide. The key role of scintillation cameras is also due to their ability to measure changes in tracer distribution as a function of time. These time-dependent changes can be quantified with a digital computer interfaced to the scintillation camera. With the hardware and software that are now available in state-of-the-art computers, special processing is commonly used to analyze data, improve image quality, and provide functional images.

The marked improvement in Anger scintillation camera performance during the past decade has not come about because of major changes in technology, but rather through a series of refinements, each of which provided a small improvement. Evolution of the Anger camera as an imaging instrument was profoundly influenced by the ready availability of technetium-99m, with its advantageous physical characteristics. Although the performance parameters of scintillation cameras will continue to improve, further advances will produce only modest improvements in the appearance of clinical images.

Physical Characteristics

The detector in an Anger scintillation camera is composed of a thin sheet of NaI(Tl) crystal, which varies from 6.4 mm (1/4 in.) to 12.7 mm (1/2 in.) in thickness and is circular, rectangular, or square in shape. The crystal is larger than the collimated field-of-view and is hermetically sealed with a thin aluminum entrance window and a glass exit window. The number of PMTs that are interfaced to the crystal varies from 37 to 91. The tubes typically are arranged in a hexagonal pattern. Increasing the number of PMTs has improved intrinsic spatial resolution by providing finer spatial sampling. Currently used PMTs are more efficient than previous varieties at converting "light" energy from the crystal into the voltage pulse used for determining both the position of a photon interaction in the crystal and the energy released by this interaction. Computers are used to control fabrication of and generate profiles on all PMTs so that they can be matched for a given camera. However, even when the tubes are "matched" and carefully balanced ("tuned"), it may still be very difficult to produce a uniform response to a flood source of radioactivity. For this and other reasons, almost all camera manufacturers have introduced special electronic circuitry that corrects for field nonuniformities. These are described in the section entitled "Correction Circuits."

The improved spatial resolution that has been seen in recent years is also a result of a decrease in detector thickness and a reduction in thickness or elimination of the light pipe. Because it can be shown that 82% of the 140-keV photons from technetium-99m are absorbed in the first 6.4 mm of the crystal, thin crystals are often used to provide improved spatial resolution with minimal loss of sensitivity for technetium-99m photons. However, the extent to which this improvement can be realized in clinical practice depends on the imaging situation. At the surface of a high-resolution collimater, the FWHM for technetium-99m decreases from 5.2 to 4.3 mm or less when the crystal thickness is reduced from 12.7 to 6.4 mm. The corresponding values for thallium-201 are 6.8 and 5.5 mm. Conversely, at 10 cm from the collimator face the FWHM decreases from 7.7 mm to only 7.6 mm for technetium-99m and from 9.2 to 8.2 mm for thallium-201. Thus, with a conventional high-resolution collimator, the change in system spatial resolution at 10 cm is probably not observable for technetium-99m; it may be for thallium-201.

As would be expected, the sensitivity decreases when thinner crystals are used. For technetium-99m (140 keV), the detector photopeak efficiency decreases from almost 100% for a crystal 12.7 mm thick to 82% for a crystal 6.4 mm thick. Thallium-201 photons (approximately 80 keV) are detected with almost 100% efficiency, even with thin crystals. In sharp contrast, only 30% of the photons from iodine-131 (364 keV) are stopped by a 12.7-mm detector of NaI(Tl). Therefore, for general clinical use, it may be appropriate to select a camera with a thicker crystal to provide better efficiency for radionuclides, such as gallium-67 and iodine-131, which have higher energy emissions. Conversely, if a camera is to be used only for imaging thallium-201 and technetium-99m, a thin crystal may be more appropriate. With the recent improvements in camera technology, most manufacturers provide either 9.5- or 12.7-mm detectors for large-field cameras.

Reduction in crystal thickness and the use of correction circuits have also produced an improvement in energy resolution from 14% to 9% for technetium-99m (Table 1). Good energy resolution is important because scattered photons can be eliminated more efficiently, and contrast and spatial resolution are improved.

Table 1
PERFORMANCE CHARACTERISTICS OF LARGE-FIELD SCINTILLATION CAMERAS

Measured parameter (^{99m}Tc)	Range of values
Intrinsic integral field uniformity*	2.0–5.4%
Intrinsic differential field uniformity*	2–5%
Intrinsic spatial resolution (FWHM)*	3.5–4.8 mm
Intrinsic energy resolution	9.8–14%
Intrinsic temporal resolution	
Maximum observed count rate	105K–325K cps
Observed count rate for 20% loss	65K–185K cps

* Central field-of-view at 20K cps. FWHM = full width at half maximum.

Position and Energy Determination

When an x-ray or gamma ray interacts with the crystal, a flash of light is produced. Each PMT "sees" some fraction of the total light that is released and generates a voltage pulse that is proportional to the intensity of this "light." An analog computer, sometimes called the position-encoding network, compares the voltage output of the PMTs and after eliminating very weak signals by thresholding, computes the position of the event using a rectilinear coordinate system. Because image size is a function of photon energy, it is also necessary to divide the X and Y signals by the photon energy. Without use of this "ratio circuit," it would not be possible to image more than one photon energy at the same time because the images would be of two different sizes. The X and Y position signals are passed to the display CRT to move the electron beam to a position on the phosphor face that corresponds to the xy position where the x-ray or gamma ray interacted with the NaI(Tl) detector. The X and Y coordinates of this event may also be simultaneously transferred to a computer. For technetium-99m, state-of-the-art scintillation cameras are capable of determining the position of individual events in the crystal to within 3 to 5 mm (FWHM) (see Table 1).

A separate circuit is used to determine the energy deposited by an individual photon. This is accomplished by adding together the voltage signals from all of the PMTs to provide one composite pulse (Z pulse). If the energy of this Z pulse meets the acceptable energy range specified by the setting on the pulse-height analyzer, (i.e., an energy level appropriate for a primary photon or a photon that has been scattered through a small angle only), an unblank signal is generated, and the electron beam on the CRT is turned on for a few microseconds or less. When a computer is interfaced to the camera, the unblank signal is also used to increment the appropriate pixel in the computer's memory by one count. The size of the analyzer window represents a compromise between a wide energy range, which would provide more counts but degrade the image resolution and contrast by accepting more scatter, and a narrow energy range, which would greatly limit the counts that can be collected for imaging in a reasonable period of time. For cameras having energy resolution between 9% and 12%, an appropriate compromise is to use 15% windows for static planar imaging and single-photon emission computed tomographic (SPECT) studies.

In some cameras, special circuits are provided to automatically position analyzer windows. The analyzer window is first split in half; then the gain is adjusted until the count rate in both halves is the same. Although this method has the advantage of being operator independent, it can create problems if the patient is used to "peak" the camera because the presence of scatter causes the window setting to be skewed to the low-energy side. The result is reduced contrast.

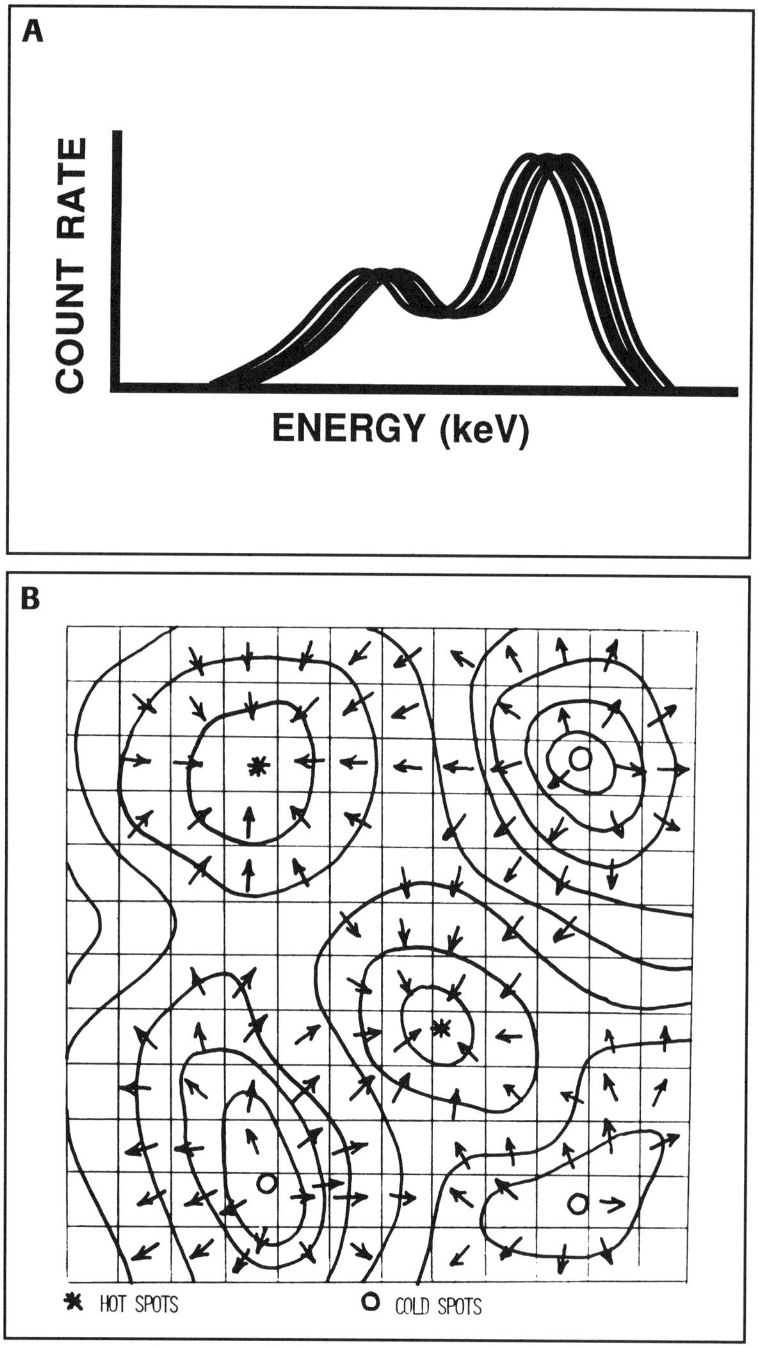

Figure 1 (A) Variations in position of the photopeak along the energy axis as a function of position on the detector surface. (B) Schematic showing production of "hot" and "cold" spots in an Anger camera because of mispositioning of individual events.

Most cameras utilize electronic formatters to provide high-resolution images that can be displayed in different formats and sizes and are capable of rapidly switching from one image position to the next to provide "flow" images. These formatters use special electronic techniques to provide small dots so that resolution is not degraded by significant overlap of individual events.

Correction Circuits

Because smaller, more efficient PMTs are used and are positioned closer to the crystal to produce improved spatial resolution, it has been necessary to install special circuits in Anger scintillation cameras to maintain a uniform response to a uniform flux of radiation. In general terms, field nonuniformity is produced by two factors. When a point source of radiation is moved to a different position on the face of a collimated detector, the position of the photopeak will shift as a result of changes in light-collection efficiency (Fig. 1A). In some locations, the center of the photopeak will be shifted toward the high-energy side; in others, toward the low-energy side. When scatter is present, an upward shift will cause the observed count rate to increase. A downward shift will produce a decrease in the observed count rate. Small changes in inherent crystal sensitivity also make a minor contribution to point source sensitivity variations. Careful measurements will also reveal that individual events are not positioned properly, that is, the camera produces distortions (nonlinearities) in positioning events (Fig. 1B). A "hot" spot is produced by the local compression of individual events; a "cold" spot is the result of local expansion.

In older cameras, onboard microprocessors were used to "skim" counts from hot areas, add counts to cold areas, or alter the unblank time on the display CRT so that a change in dot intensity would compensate for regional variations in counts observed in a uniform flood. Such techniques produced cosmetic changes only and did not correct the underlying errors. Now, almost all state-of-the-art scintillation cameras use more elaborate and sophisticated techniques to produce uniform images while maintaining high spatial resolution.

Correction for shifts of the photopeak in different locations on the detector (energy or Z correction) begins with careful measurement of changes in the location of the photopeak over the entire useful field of the detector: 128 × 128 or 256 × 256 matrices are usually used for this purpose. Once the shifts of the photopeak have been measured for each location, correction maps are prepared and stored in a microprocessor. When images are acquired, individual events are corrected by shifting the window to its appropriate position relative to the photopeak or adjusting the voltage of the Z pulse so that it is positioned correctly relative to a fixed window (Fig. 2A).

Correction for distortion (nonlinearity) is accomplished in a similar way. Distortions are carefully measured using a fine matrix, and correction factors are computed. These distortion correction maps are stored in a microprocessor, and individual events are repositioned as an image is acquired (Fig. 2B).

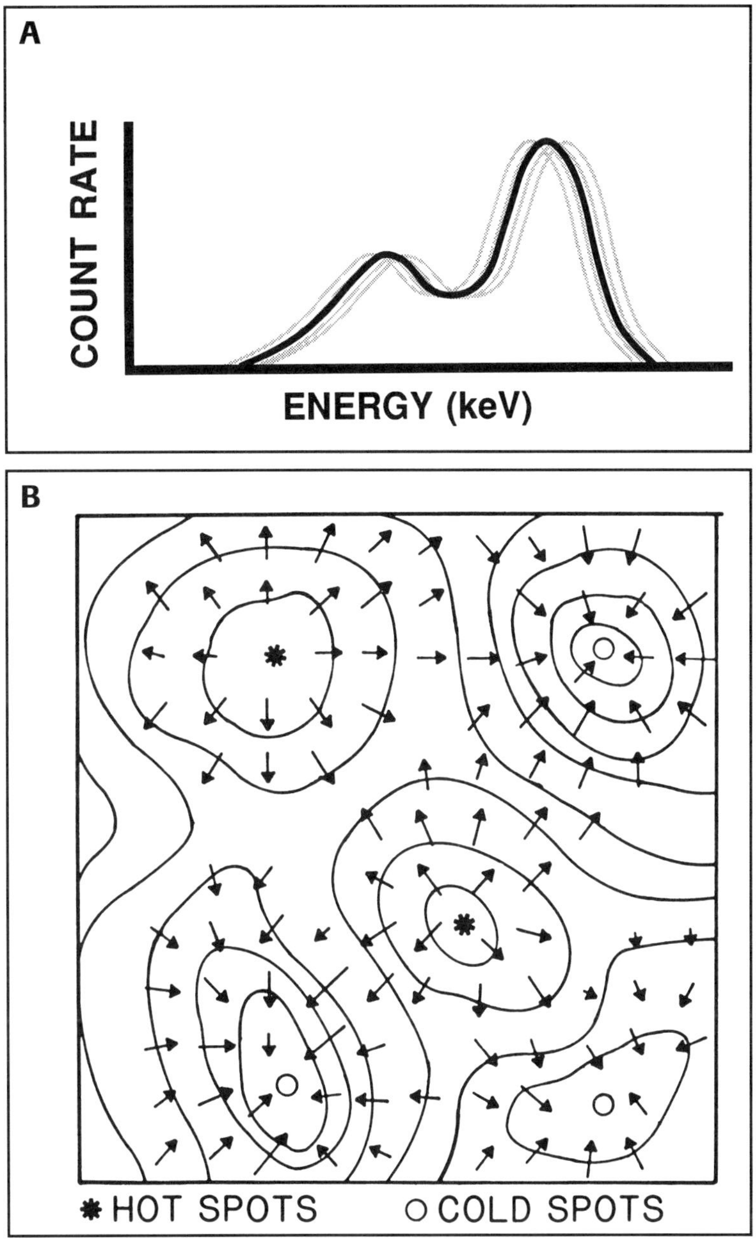

Figure 2 (A) Schematic of composite spectrum after application of energy correction. (B) Schematic showing repositioning of individual events to correct for distortion (nonlinearity).

When the energy and distortion correction circuits are working properly, and the camera is properly tuned, excellent field uniformity is obtained. The availability of energy correction circuitry also makes possible the use of asymmetric windows without the introduction of artifacts. Positioning the analyzer window slightly to the high side of the photopeak improves spatial resolution. It is well known that when technetium-99m is used, the scatter part of the spectrum overlaps the photopeak on the low-energy side (Fig. 3). If an asymmetric window is set so that more of the upper part of the photopeak is included, fewer scattered photons will be used in the image-formation process. The final result is an image with improved spatial resolution and contrast, especially for deep-lying structures. In general, asymmetric windows should not be used on cameras without an energy correction circuit because nonuniformities may appear. Even in cameras that utilize energy correction circuitry, there is a limit to the degree of asymmetry that can be tolerated without introducing artifacts into the corrected image. Before asymmetric windows are used clinically, the uniformity must be evaluated as a function of asymmetry.

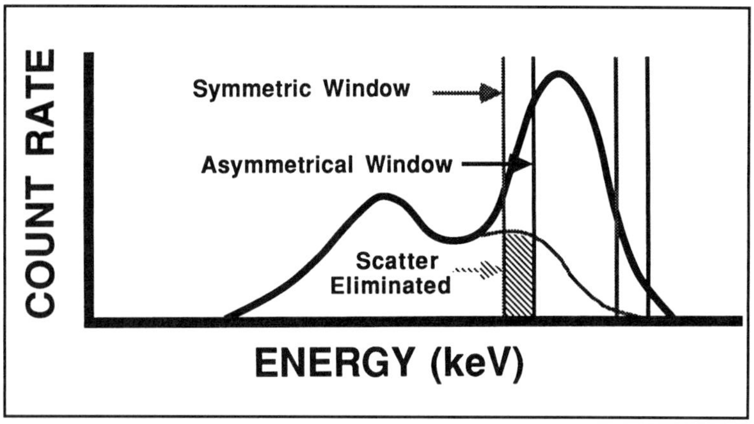

Figure 3 Schematic showing reduction of scatter in the analyzer window by use of asymmetric high windows for technetium-99m.

Energy and distortion correction maps are prepared on cameras that do not have a collimator in place, that is, they are prepared intrinsically. As a result, nonuniformities that are due to variations in the response of the collimator may still be present. In some cameras it is also possible to generate and save a sensitivity map for each collimator. Correction for collimator nonuniformities can then be applied after a study is completed. This final correction, which can also be done using an external computer, also corrects for any global variations in camera response that are a function of photon energy. In other words, sensitivity maps for different radionuclides can also be stored.

Automatic Tuning

Because the energy and distortion correction maps are prepared when the PMTs are properly balanced, it is imperative that the camera be maintained in a properly tuned state; otherwise, the use of correction circuitry may result in a worse camera response than if correction circuits were not used. Unfortunately, even under the best of conditions all PMTs exhibit varying gain shifts over time. Most Anger cameras now contain special circuits that automatically adjust the high voltage or amplifier gain to maintain PMT balance. Several different techniques are used for automatic tuning.

Two commercially produced camera systems use light-emitting diodes (LEDs) to check the gain of each PMT. When the LED is flashed, the light causes the PMT to generate a voltage pulse. Either the individual pulse or a short-term running average of the voltage (approximately 1 sec) is compared to a reference value and the gain of the PMT adjusted, if necessary. One significant difference between the techniques that are used by these two manufacturers should be noted: On one camera the LED is flashed many times per second (even while an image is being collected); on the other, the tuning sequence is performed before clinical studies are begun. The former was developed to correct for changes in camera uniformity during SPECT studies because of the effect of the earth's magnetic field on PMT signal output.

Two different camera systems use radiation from radionuclides to tune the camera automatically. Pulse height analyzer windows are used to monitor the location of the photopeak, and PMT gain is adjusted, if necessary. One of the systems performs this operation during the clinical imaging process; the other balances the PMTs on demand.

One other technique is currently used for automatic tuning. The actual high voltage on each PMT is monitored and compared to a set of reference values. If the values do not agree to within a specific tolerance, the voltage is automatically adjusted.

There is no question that the availability of automatic tuning techniques has significantly improved the performance of Anger cameras. However, this improved performance does not eliminate or reduce the need for a comprehensive quality control and preventative maintenance program.

Scatter Reduction

Until recently, scintillation cameras have utilized one to four pulse height analyzer windows to select the primary unscattered photons and those that have been scattered through relatively small angles. By necessity, the analyzer window size and position have been chosen as a compromise between rejecting all scattered photons at the expense of decreased statistics and accepting some scattered photons at the expense of decreasing contrast. At this time a number of vendors have incorporated hardware and software into current cameras that reduce or "eliminate" scatter. Most are based on the use of narrow pulse height analyzer windows on a pixel-by-pixel basis to determine the shape of the spectrum and separate scatter from photopeak events. While there are some variations in their effectiveness, all of the techniques provide improved contrast at the cost of some increase in noise. This is a common tradeoff that must be made in image processing.

	-0.0247	-0.0247	-0.0247	
-0.0247	+0.0182	+0.1270	+0.0182	-0.0247
-0.0247	+0.1270	+0.5849	+0.1270	-0.0247
-0.0247	+0.0182	+0.1270	+0.0182	-0.0247
	-0.0247	-0.0247	-0.0247	

Figure 4 Example of one of the spatial filters used for scatter removal by energy-weighted acquisition (EWA).

Count Rate Performance

A fundamental principle of nuclear medicine is that a change in the activity in an organ or region is reflected as an increase or decrease in the number of observed counts. Unfortunately, scintillation cameras do not respond linearly to an increase in activity throughout the range of activities that are normally administered. Up to 20 mCi, most state-of-the-art Anger cameras follow a paralyzable model, as represented by the following equation:

$$R(\text{true}) = R(\text{obs}) * \exp[R(\text{true}) * t(\text{par})],$$

where R(true) is the true count rate; R(obs) is the observed count rate; and t(par) is the paralyzable resolving time. This model predicts that when a camera is exposed to increasing amounts of radiation, a maximum count rate will be reached beyond which the count rate will actually decrease. It is generally recommended that clinical studies should not be performed if the difference between the observed count rate and a linear response (no coincidence losses) is greater than 27%. At this point, a 2% increase in activity produces only a 1% increase in the observed count rate.

In recent years, a number of techniques have been developed to improve the count rate performance of scintillation cameras. One involves the use of derandomizer buffers. These devices consist of electronic slots where subsequent events can be temporarily saved while a previous event is being processed. Derandomizer buffers usually have from three to six stages and are appropriate because of the random nature of radioactive decay.

If two randomly occurring gamma-ray events occur within a time equal to the integration (light collection) time, the second pulse is said to be "piled up" on the first. When this occurs, both pulses are rejected to avoid distortion of the signal. Many modern cameras have pileup rejection circuits. Pulses that become "piled up" do not appear to decay as rapidly and can be rejected at an earlier stage. Time is not wasted in pulse-height analysis, and count rate performance is improved.

Count rate performance has also been improved by adding a second integrator. The time that is required to transfer the output from the integrator to the display and reset the integrator is longer than the normal integration time. Thus, if an event occurs during the transfer and reset time, it is rejected. When there are two integrator circuits, they can alternately integrate and transfer signals. As a result, count rate performance is improved without loss of spatial resolution.

Count rate performance can also be improved by installing a special switch that alters the method by which signals are processed. In simple terms, this modification decreases the time during which light is collected from the crystal (integration time). In some systems, the pileup rejection criteria are also relaxed. Because individual signals are processed more rapidly, the probability of coincidence at high counting rates (pulse pileup) is reduced, but there is an accompanying loss of spatial resolution. However, because this mode of operation is only used when the counting rate is high, usually for first-pass cardiac studies where statistics are poor, any loss of spatial resolution is more than offset by the improvement in statistics. In some cameras, selection of the "fast" mode disables the energy and linearity correction circuits.

Motion Correction

It is well known that images are degraded in the presence of object motion. Several different approaches have been used to minimize its effect on radionuclide images of the liver, lung, and heart. An electronic gate can be used to acquire images only during a part of the respiration cycle. Alternatively, a computer can be used to correct for organ motion retrospectively. However, analog circuit techniques are attractive because they are inexpensive and do not require computer time. The X and Y positioning circuits are integrated over a short time interval to provide a signal that is proportional to the centroid. When the centroid changes, a bias is applied to the deflection circuits of the image display to reposition the image relative to the center of the detector. The end result is to hold the centroid in a fixed position. Studies have confirmed the clinical utility of motion correction in liver imaging.

Another approach to motion correction involves the use of two different radionuclides. A point source of americum-241 taped to the skin is used as a reference marker and is imaged using a second analyzer window. Data from the second window are integrated at short time intervals, and the location of the centroid is used to reposition the image in the primary window. Data suggest that this technique may be helpful in correcting for motion when a gated wall motion study of the heart is recorded during exercise.

Digital Circuitry and Smart Consoles

The widespread availability of microprocessors has led to the introduction of "smart" consoles and "digital" cameras. When the "smart console" is used, all camera functions are set from a keyboard. This makes possible the use of preset protocols for clinical studies, thus increasing throughput and reproducibility of studies. In addition, microprocessors can be used to adjust the display for different types of film, place annotation on the film, and provide the variations of image display commonly seen in minicomputers (i.e., background subtraction, contrast enhancement). Microprocessors can also process data to produce time–activity curves and analyze gated wall motion studies.

Digital cameras have evolved as many of the electronic subsystems have been replaced by computer software. When modifications are required, the electronics need not be redesigned; instead, the algorithms can be changed to accommodate the required modification. As the cost of digital components decreases, more and more manufacturers will incorporate them for economic reasons. Because analog components and circuitry are still used for the early stages of signal processing, including the position-encoding circuits, a truly digital camera does not yet exist.

Collimators

Several developments have occurred in the field of collimation that have improved clinical performance. Probably the most important advance has been the introduction of "foil" collimators. They are made by laminating thin (7–15 mils) corrugated strips of lead. State-of-the-art collimators utilize hexagonal holes in a hexagonal pattern. This design offers the best combination of sensitivity and resolution of any hole pattern and provides more sensitivity than circular hole, cast collimators with the same spatial resolution. The increased sensitivity can be used to improve statistics for first-pass or exercise wall motion studies and to decrease imaging time in general.

MULTIPLE-ELEMENT SCINTILLATION CAMERA

An alternative approach to the use of a thin, large-diameter crystal is to use a single block of NaI(Tl) divided into small detector elements. The Scinticor camera contains 400 elements in a 20 × 20 matrix. Individual segments are surrounded by reflective material, and the array is viewed directly by 115 PMTs (light pipes are not used). Each scintillation activates only two PMTs so that positioning is independent of pulse height analysis, and very high count rates can be achieved. Although spatial resolution and energy resolution are not as good as that for Anger cameras, count rates of 650,000 to 870,000 cps have been recorded for 15–30 mCi of technetium-99m using a wide-open analyzer window. In addition, spatial resolution does not deteriorate at high count rates. Hence, this camera offers two important advantages over Anger camera technology for first-transit studies obtained with technetium-99m and gold-195m.

EFFECT OF CAMERA PERFORMANCE ON CLINICAL IMAGING

It has been clearly established that for both planar and ECT imaging, poor field uniformity of the scintillation camera leads to an increase in the false positive rate for lesion detection. The actual uniformity that is required for optimum image quality depends on a large number of factors, including count density, image size, type of display media, type of study (hot- or cold-spot imaging), and contrast. In SPECT imaging, good field uniformity is particularly important because errors caused by nonuniformities are exaggerated by the reconstruction process.

Although a high degree of spatial resolution may not be necessary to perform studies embodying the tracer principle, good resolution is useful for most clinical imaging situations. It must be appreciated that spatial resolution of the scintillation camera system as a whole is determined by the following relation:

$$R_{sys} = \sqrt{R^2_{intrin} + R_{coll} + R^2_{scat}},$$

where R_{intrin} is the intrinsic spatial resolution; R_{coll} is the collimator resolution; and R_{scat} is the scatter resolution. Large improvements in intrinsic resolution beyond that of state-of-the-art cameras will not have a dramatic effect on system resolution because of the limiting effects of collimator resolution and scatter. A study of planar liver and bone imaging documented that when intrinsic resolution was lowered from 4.9 to 3.7 mm, no significant improvement in image quality could be seen. However, gains in intrinsic resolution assist the detection of superficial lesions because for these lesions, system resolution is less dependent on collimator performance.

The high degree of intrinsic spatial resolution provided by state-of-the-art cameras may present a problem when medium-energy collimators are used. Moiré patterns can be seen to distort bar-pattern images but have not been reported in clinical studies. These patterns are due to the interplay between the lead septa of the collimator and the cyclic variations in the bar pattern and may be of importance in the interpretation of quality control images.

Spatial resolution and contrast can be improved by the use of asymmetrically placed analyzer windows. Because scatter events fall on the low side of the photopeak, positioning the window slightly to the right of center (high side) improves the quality of information (ratio of unscattered to scattered photons) used to compose clinical images. However, this advantage is partially offset by a decrease in the number of counts obtained per unit time. In some cameras, asymmetrically positioned windows also produce a loss of uniformity.

From the standpoint of clinical imaging, several general points about collimators should be kept in mind:

1. Foil collimators require special care because of their fragile nature. They can easily be damaged during shipment and should be carefully tested at the time of installation. In addition, they can be damaged by rough handling and should be checked periodically as a part of a quality control program. Collimator defects can produce artifacts in clinical studies.

2. Slant-hole collimators provide better spatial resolution than conventional parallel-hole collimators because they allow the collimator face to be positioned closer to the patient, but the resultant images show an ellipsoid distortion of the target organ. Many clinicians consider that the improvement in spatial resolution offsets the distortion that is present. Improved system resolution shows up in cardiac studies as more clearly delineated edges. System spatial resolution is a more important factor in the evaluation of regional cardiac wall motion than it is for the task of lesion detection. The slant-hole collimator can also be used for hepatobiliary scans, evaluation of vertebral–body abnormalities, and obtaining caudal and cephalad views of the posterior fossa and rib, pubic bone, and sacral bone lesions.

3. Converging collimators have several properties that make them particularly useful in clinical imaging. Because they magnify the image, system resolution can approach that of the uncollimated detector at the expense of field-of-view. In addition, spatial resolution falls off less rapidly with dis-

tance for converging collimators than for any other type. Although some distortion is present, it is generally considered that physicians do not have any difficulty in interpreting the images.

Count rate performance is of particular interest in certain types of clinical studies (e.g., first-pass cardiac studies for estimating right or left ventricular function). Count rate performance is also important for studies using short-lived radionuclides such as gold-195m and krypton-81m.

During studies that require 20 mCi of technetium-99m and a moderately high-efficiency collimator, as many as 400,000 photons may interact with the crystal per second. In a typical gated study with the same amount of activity, the number of photon interactions is approximately 60,000/second. The observed count rate is usually on the order of one-third of the incident count rate, but the camera must process all events to reject the invalid two-thirds. The analysis of events takes time, partly because of the time required to convert information contained in the light of the scintillation event into electronic pulses and partly because of the time needed to analyze these pulses and to record information for use in creating the image. The time during which the camera is unable to handle another event is called the "dead" or resolving time. All events incident on the crystal contribute to the dead time.

Although counts are lost when pileup occurs, the more serious problem associated with pulse pileup is the loss of spatial resolution. This occurs when two low-energy photons (e.g., scattered photons) strike the detector at nearly the same time so that their light production appears as a single event with an energy equal to the sum of their energies. Image degradation occurs when the summed energy equals the energy of an "acceptable" event because it is assigned a position that is somewhere between the position of the two individual photon interactions. The result is a "misplaced" event. Unfortunately, corrections for misplaced events and count losses are very difficult because the effect of pileup varies with the geometric distribution of the sources and the amount of scattering.

It is important to remember that with the use of currently available PMT and NaI(Tl) detectors there are limitations on what can be done to improve count rate performance. This is a consequence of the fundamental nature of fluorescence in the crystal and the characteristics of the PMT. However, recent work has shown that the limitation caused by the decay of light in the NaI(Tl) crystal has not been reached. Therefore, it seems likely that further advances in the count rate capabilities of Anger cameras will occur in the next few years.

Almost all large-field Anger scintillation cameras now have two or three analyzer windows. A single computer image can be produced from the output of all three windows, or two different images can be formed from the output of separate analyzer windows. The increase in sensitivity for gallium-67, indium-111, and thallium-201 is an illustration of the usefulness of this option. However, incorrect alignment of the images from the two (or three) different windows, called energy misregistration (multiple-window spatial registration), can seriously degrade spatial resolution, decrease contrast, and increase spatial distortion.

QUALITY CONTROL FOR ANGER CAMERAS

Quality control procedures are an essential part of quality assurance in nuclear medicine. Several organizations have provided protocols that can be followed in

Table 2
QUALITY CONTROL FOR SCINTILLATION CAMERAS

Parameter to be tested	Frequency
Analyzer calibration	Each day of use and after each change of radionuclide
Field uniformity	Each day of use
Spatial resolution and linearity	Weekly
Maximum count rate	Quarterly
Collimator uniformity	Quarterly
Multiple-window spatial registration (energy registration)	Quarterly
Sensitivity	Quarterly

performing and evaluating these tests. The types of tests and their frequency are listed in Table 2.

On a less frequent basis (e.g., semiannually), additional tests should be performed on scintillation cameras as a part of a comprehensive quality assurance program. These are presented in Table 2. Protocols for most of these tests can be found in the reference section.

A good quality assurance program should also include a preventive maintenance program that has been found to be cost-effective. This should include inspection and cleaning of equipment and replacement of items that are worn. Such a program may prevent unexpected breakdowns and disruption of service.

Conclusion

Anger scintillation cameras will probably continue to be the imaging instrument of choice for some time. Several groups are working on detectors using solid-state and image-intensifier detectors, but such instruments may be difficult to manufacture and are likely to be expensive. Efforts to further increase intrinsic resolution are probably not warranted because in most imaging situations, the collimator and the presence of scatter limit the spatial resolution that can be achieved. Therefore, it seems logical that the focus of further development should be on other aspects of camera performance.

Most practitioners agree that the principal need in nuclear medicine is a higher count rate for image production without an increase in radiation dose to the patient. What changes can be made to accomplish this goal? Further decreases in dead-time losses would be helpful for first-pass studies and for imaging with short-lived radionuclides. Faster cameras would be particularly important if changes in collimator technology provide higher sensitivity. This might come about through the use of different materials such as tantalum. Higher count rates may also be achieved through the use of faster crystals such as cesium fluoride or a return to thicker NaI(Tl) crystals, or both. The future could also bring more efficient PMTs or even replacement of PMTs with a mosaic of photodiodes to create a truly digital camera.

EMISSION COMPUTED TOMOGRAPHIC IMAGING

Single-Photon Emission Computed Tomographic Imaging

Overview. Single-photon emission computed tomographic imaging has several important advantages over planar imaging:

1. The most important advantage of SPECT imaging is that transverse section images have higher contrast than planar images. In planar imaging, overlying and underlying activity often obscures areas of decreased uptake, particularly in organ studies such as liver imaging. Transverse sections are

reconstructed through the organ, thus restoring the original high contrast by elimination of interference from overlying and underlying activity.

2. With rotating-camera systems particularly, a volume of activity is reconstructed with approximately equal resolution in all three dimensions. This allows subsequent reslicing of the distribution to permit visualization in transverse, sagittal, and coronal sections (useful in brain and liver imaging) and in oblique sections (useful in cardiac imaging). The human eye–brain combination is very good at perceiving contours and changes in image intensity that are close to each other. Therefore, a particular anatomic structure may be easily perceived in the sagittal view, whereas another may be better visualized in the transverse section.
3. Single-photon emission computed tomographic imaging can aid in quantitation. Clearly, if the activity is reconstructed as a true three-dimensional distribution, the measured intensity is more easily related to the true radioisotope concentration than in planar imaging, where overlying and underlying activity and background activity often interfere.

The introduction of SPECT imaging into routine clinical nuclear medicine is taking a long time, due in part to the fact that early SPECT systems were generally of poor quality. It took several years for instrumentation manufacturers to invest the necessary resources to develop SPECT systems that gave artifact-free, high-resolution reconstructed images. Single-photon emission computed tomographic imaging not only improves the contrast of images depicting the radioisotope distribution in the patient, but also enhances image distortions caused by imperfections in the imaging system. Therefore, the requirements for instrumentation quality are much more rigorous for SPECT systems than for planar imaging devices. Very often scintillation cameras that provide perfectly acceptable planar images prove to be inadequate for SPECT imaging.

There are many sources of potential problems, including the influence of the earth's magnetic field on the PMT response during camera rotation, differences between the mechanical center of rotation and the center of rotation assumed in the reconstruction algorithm, collimator imperfections, and spatial distortions in the scintillation detector. These problems usually cause either reduced spatial resolution or circular artifacts centered on the center of rotation of the camera. To avoid or correct for these problems, modern, good-quality SPECT systems are provided with good magnetic shielding around the PMTs, spatial linearity correction, spatially varying energy windows, and procedures for uniformity and center-of-rotation correction. Although improved instrumentation makes it significantly easier to take good-quality SPECT images, stringent quality control is necessary to obtain high-resolution artifact-free images. This requires more time for quality control and additional service calls to keep the instrument performing well. Furthermore, positioning the patient is still difficult because one must ensure that the rotating scintillation camera does not hit the patient. However, if performed conscientiously, SPECT imaging is well worth the extra time and care because of its excellent diagnostic accuracy.

Recent Advances in Rotating-Camera Systems: Elliptic Orbit. Obviously, the simplest mechanical motion for a rotating camera is circular. Unfortunately, circular motion implies that the detectors will often be at a significant distance from the surface of the patient, particularly when the patient has a slim torso. Because resolution degrades nearly linearly with distance from the face of the collimator, this increased distance results in loss of spatial resolution. Many SPECT systems now have the capability to travel in a noncircular orbit by either raising and lowering the patient bed while the detector describes a circular motion or by moving the detector assembly of the scintillation camera during rotation. The particular choice of corrective motion may result in an orbit that is not exactly elliptic; but so long as the reconstruction software corrects for the motion of either the bed or the camera, the transverse section images thus obtained have better contrast and resolution than tomographic images from circular orbit systems.

Data Collection for Cardiac Imaging. Cardiac imaging represents a challenge for SPECT imaging, particularly when performed with thallium-201. Not only is the body contour typically elliptic, but the organ of interest, the heart, is not located at the center of rotation. This is of significance because it is imperative that the organ of interest be within the field-of-view of the scintillation camera in all views. Furthermore, the low energy of thallium-201 emissions results in significant attenuation so that few meaningful data are collected when the patient is imaged from the side opposite the heart. For this reason, 180° data collection is typically used in cardiac imaging. Dual-head SPECT systems with the heads positioned at 90° relative to each other provide the highest efficiency. Data collection is started at 45° to the right anterior, with the center of rotation of the camera positioned near the center of the heart. However, attenuation correction is more difficult in 180° than in 360° data collection. Also, some argue that artifacts are more common when data are collected only over 180°.

Special Configurations for Brain Imaging. High-resolution brain imaging presents a particular problem because of interference between the shoulders and the camera housing. If the chosen radius of rotation is large enough to avoid the shoulders, there will be a serious loss in spatial resolution due to the large distance between the face of the collimator and the brain. Although some cameras have been carefully designed to minimize the distance from the edge of the housing to the beginning of the useful field-of-view, thereby permitting clearance of the shoulders while keeping all of the brain within the field-of-view, some designs have been modified to allow the camera housing to clear the shoulders.

If a slant-hole collimator is used, the camera head can be tilted to avoid the patient's shoulders while keeping the face of the collimator close to the patient's head. A slant-hole collimator allows the use of existing reconstruction algorithms, which assume that sets of projections can be associated with a single plane without contamination from adjacent planes. This occurs when the slant angle of the holes equals the tilt angle of the camera.

Fan-Beam and Cone-Beam Collimation. When a small organ such as the brain is imaged with a large field-of-view scintillation camera, most of the crystal area is not utilized for data collection. To increase the area of the scintillation crystal that is used, and thereby increase the sensitivity and/or spatial resolution, one can use fan-beam collimators in which the collimator holes are focused in the transverse plane but continue to be at right angles to the axis of rotation (Fig. 5A). In this case, the reconstruction algorithms that were originally developed for fan-beam x-ray computed tomographic (CT) scanners can be used, but the collimator preserves the important quality that projections may still be associated with specific transverse planes without projections crossing from one plane to the next.

More recently, reconstruction algorithms have been developed that elegantly solve the problem for imaging situations in which projections are not restricted to lie in parallel planes, thereby making it possible to use two-dimensional converging collimators (Fig. 5B) to increase sensitivity and spatial resolution even further. The holes in such a collimator may either focus to a single point (cone-beam collimators) or converge to different points in the axial and transverse directions (astigmatic collimators). Using either of these collimators together with the appropriate reconstruction algorithm results in sensitivity approximately three times better than that provided by a parallel-hole collimator of comparable spatial resolution. Although these collimators can definitely be used for brain imaging, continued research will be necessary before they can be successfully applied to cardiac imaging, where peripheral activity in organs such as the liver presents additional problems.

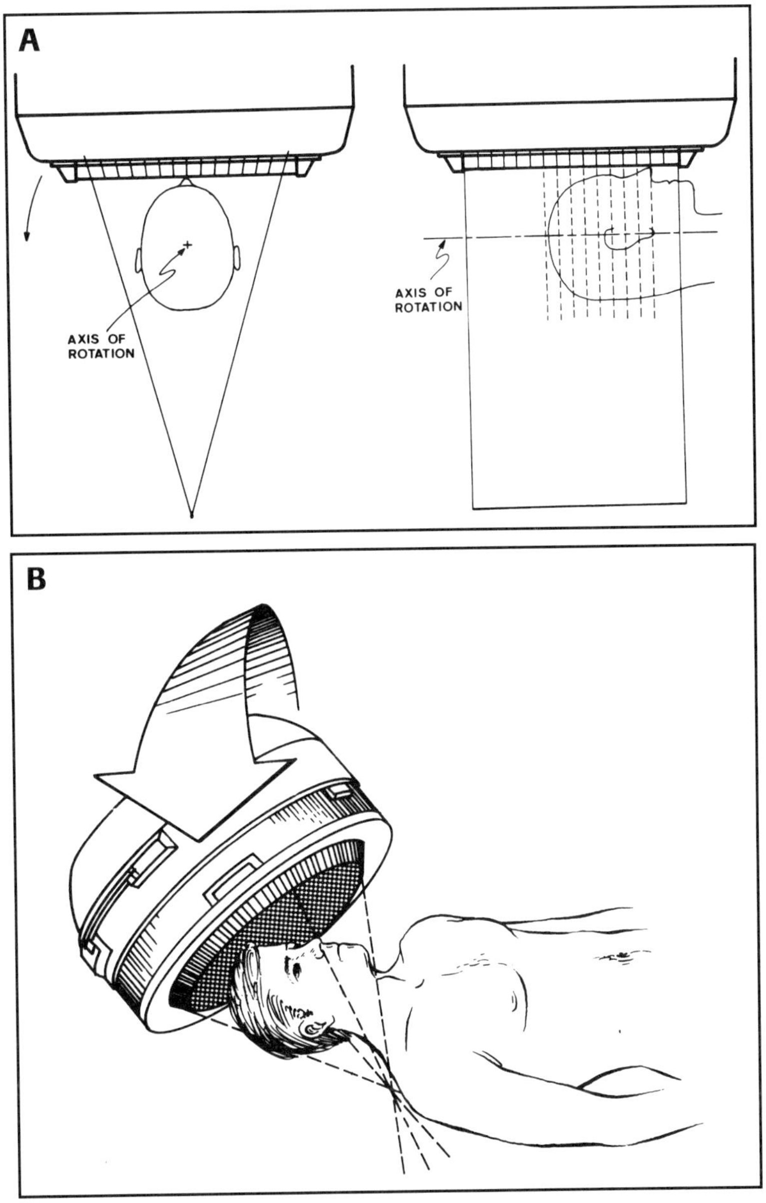

Figure 5 (A) Geometry for fan-beam collimation in transverse and axial directions. (B) Single-photon emission computed tomographic imaging of the brain with cone-beam collimator (Courtesy of Dr. R.J. Jaszczak, Duke University.)

Volume Smoothing. If the image from a large field-of-view camera with a useful diameter of 400 mm is digitized in a 128 × 128 matrix, then each pixel is approximately 3 mm × 3 mm; and if such a system is used in SPECT imaging, each slice will be 3 mm thick. Because the spatial resolution of a collimated Anger camera is much worse than 3 mm (typically 7–10 mm), the spatial sampling is less than one-half of the resolution. This is appropriate because the sampling theorem predicts that little information is lost if samples are taken at one-half to one-third of the FWHM resolution. The advantage of thin slices (even though the spatial resolution may be 7 or 10 mm) is that it is relatively easy to select a slice that is centered on a target region in the transverse plane. Such plane selection minimizes partial volume effects.

The disadvantage of thin slices, however, is the limited statistical accuracy of the data in each slice. Because the collected data are distributed over so many thin slices, each slice has poor statistical accuracy, resulting in noisy reconstructions. Smoothing in both the axial and transverse directions (i.e., volume smoothing) reduces the statistical fluctuations in all three dimensions while preserving the advantage of closely spaced slices. It is important to be aware of the fact that both limited axial resolution and smoothing in the axial direction have the effect of giving overlapping rather than contiguous slices.

Reslicing at Arbitrary Angles. Although organs such as the brain are adequately viewed in transverse, sagittal, and coronal slices, it is sometimes advantageous to be able to reslice the three-dimensionally measured radioisotope distribution at an arbitrary angle. Such oblique angle reconstruction is especially valuable in cardiac imaging. Most SPECT software programs, therefore, have provisions to sample the three-dimensional data in an arbitrary plane so that one can construct images at right angles to the major axis of the heart. In this projection it is easier for the observer to detect abnormal patterns in the distribution of the radiopharmaceutical.

Attenuation Correction. Without attenuation correction, reconstructed images will show increased signal intensity along the periphery and decreased intensity toward the center of the body because gamma radiation originating near the center of the patient has a higher probability of being scattered or absorbed. To perform accurate attenuation correction, it is necessary to know the specific attenuation coefficient for each unit volume of tissue within a transverse section. Because such information is rarely available, it is usually assumed that the attenuation coefficient is constant throughout the slice, which is reasonable for brain imaging but not for sections that include heart, lungs, and chest wall. Even if it is assumed that the attenuation coefficient is constant, it is still necessary to determine the body contour. The simplest way is to visually fit an ellipse around the image reconstructed without attenuation correction and then perform the attenuation correction by assuming a constant attenuation coefficient within the elliptic outline. Frequently, the outline of the body can be seen on the projection data so that it is also possible to indicate the body contour on the projections. However, this may be more time-consuming because the body contour must be marked on many projection views.

In the last few years, several techniques have been developed to correct for nonuniform attentuation in the chest. One method involves placing a line source of Gd-153, or other appropriate radionuclide, opposite one of the detectors on a triple-head system. All of the detectors have fan beam collimators. During the SPECT study, two detectors collect emission data while the third head acquires the transmission data. Data from the transmission scan are reconstructed to produce an attenuation map which is used to correct the emission images. An alternative technique is commonly used on dual-head SPECT systems. An apparatus is attached to each head that moves a line source of radiation over the patient at the same time the emission data are collected. As with the fan beam method, the reconstructed attentuation map is used to correct the emission data. Clinical data demonstrate an improvement in specificity when nonuniform attenuation correction is used, but recent studies indicate that the best results are obtained when scatter correction is used in conjunction with attenuation correction.

Finally, the body contour can be determined automatically by placing a second energy window well below the photopeak where most of the detected radiation represents photons that have been scattered in the body. The body contours are then well delineated, and automatic edge-finding algorithms can be used to determine the body contour from which attenuation factors can be calculated with the assumption of a constant attenuation coefficient.

Dual- and Triple-Headed Imaging Systems. It is obvious that maximum sensitivity can be obtained if the patient is completely surrounded by detectors. This ideal can be reasonably approximated if three scintillation cameras are arranged triangularly, particularly if the cameras are equipped with fan-beam collimators so that the whole crystal area is utilized. Using two scintillation cameras is a compromise that nearly achieves the sensitivity of a three-headed system, with the added advantage that the system may be used for simultaneous collection of anterior and posterior planar images in organ studies requiring both views, such as bone and liver imaging. A number of vendors offer dual-head cameras with a 90° configuration. In some systems, the detectors are fixed; in others the heads can be rotated to 90° from the 180° configuration. The improved sensitivity can be traded for shorter imaging time and higher patient throughput, improved image quality, or lower radionuclide dose with reduced radiation exposure to the patient. Quality control problems, however, increase with a multiheaded rotating Anger camera system because all detector heads must not only have the same center of rotation, but their linearity must be matched so that data from all detector heads can be summed without loss of spatial resolution.

Dedicated SPECT Scanners. *Cylindrical camera-based systems.* The fact that the best scanner performance is achieved if the patient is completely surrounded by scintillation detectors has led to the development of some novel and potentially useful configurations. In one approach, a large number of PMTs are mounted on the outer surface of a single cylindrical scintillation crystal. This method has the advantage of mechanical simplicity because the detector can be kept stationary; the only rotating component is a cylindrical collimator positioned against the inner surface of the crystal. However, a large cylindrical scintillation crystal is somewhat expensive, and any failure due to thermal stress, physical impact, or broken hermetic seal would result in a major expense. A similar approach, pursued by Rogers et al. at the University of Michigan, replaces the single cylindrical crystal with several smaller position-sensitive detectors. This design retains the advantage of a stationary detector but avoids the risk associated with a single cylindrical crystal. However, with either approach, the crystal diameter must be selected either for brain or body imaging. A system designed for body imaging would not be optimal for brain imaging because the detectors would be too far from the organ.

At the time that SPECT imaging was introduced into routine clinical nuclear medicine, it was important to justify the equipment purchase with the argument that a rotating-camera system could also perform planar studies. At many institutions, enough SPECT studies are now being performed to justify a dedicated SPECT imaging system, and systems with a stationary detector have some significant advantages over rotating-camera systems. Conversely, cylindrical stationary detector systems will not have an elliptic orbit because the collimator must rotate, resulting in some loss of spatial resolution compared to a rotating-camera system. It should be noted that the three-headed rotating Anger camera system preserves the elliptic orbit while at the same time surrounding the patient with detectors from practically all sides.

Multicrystal Scanners. More than 10 years ago, a dedicated SPECT system became commercially available (Cleon/Union Carbide Corporation) and came to be known as the Harvard scanner after Union Carbide abandoned it. It has recently been redesigned and is again commercially available (Strickman). This scanner incorporates 12 large crystals (8 in. × 5 in. × 1 in.) that are focused onto a single slice, so that the sensitivity is extremely high in that slice. To scan an organ completely, it is necessary to perform many contiguous or overlapping scans. Thus, while the imaging time per slice is quite short, a complete study takes approximately the same time as it does with a camera-based system.

Published reports are full of conflicting claims about the relative advantages and disadvantages of camera-based and multicrystal SPECT systems. A short description of some of their differences and their potential impact on clinical performance is therefore appropriate. Figure 6A illustrates the differences in the two approaches in the axial direction. A rotating-camera system is typically

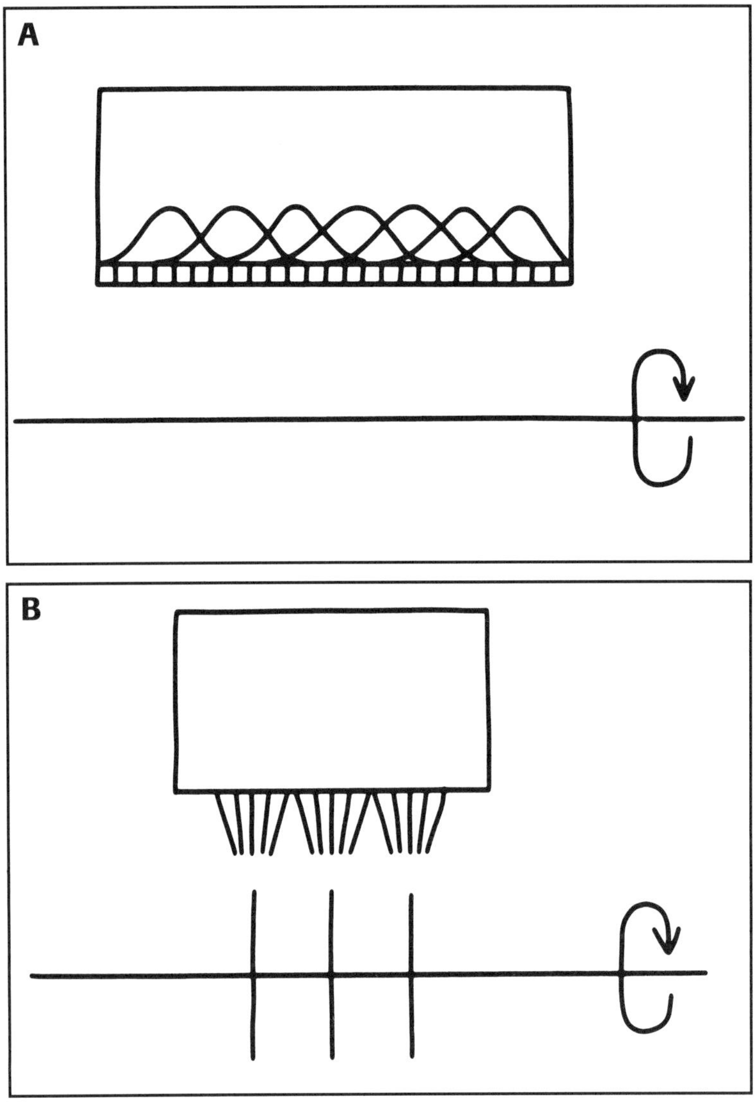

Figure 6 (A) Axial collimation in rotating Anger camera system typically samples the object continuously as well as with overlapping slices. (B) In a multicrystal scanner, sensitivity is usually concentrated in a few slices with gaps. This results in higher slice sensitivity but requires axial scanning for complete organ coverage.

equipped with a parallel-hole collimator, or at least a collimator with holes parallel in the axial direction (fanbeam). Thus, the entire volume of the organ of interest is under observation at all times, and data are collected for all slices simultaneously such that both contiguous and overlapping slices can be obtained. In a multicrystal scanner approach, as illustrated in Figure 6B, the sensitivity is collimated to focus on one or several slices such that these slices are imaged at very high sensitivity; but if one wishes to study the whole organ, multiple slices are necessary.

Theoretically, it is immaterial whether all slices are observed simultaneously at reduced sensitivity in a single scan or whether a few slices are observed at high sensitivity but require multiple repetitions. Both methods require the same scanning time so long as the axial crystal dimension is the same. This point is critical—if the detector is extended in the axial direction and the collimator holes are angled to focus the sensitivity to an organ with a limited axial extent, then a true increase in sensitivity can be obtained, as exemplified by the cone-beam or astigmatic collimator.

The two approaches for the transverse direction are compared in Figure 7. To obtain artifact-free ECT reconstructions, it is necessary to observe every point in the transverse plane from all directions. This is achieved with a rotating camera equipped with a parallel-hole collimator that collects all the data at one angle simultaneously and then, as a function of time, collects the data from all other angles. This is in contrast to the multicrystal scanner, which observes all angles simultaneously because each of the 12 detectors has approximately a 30° acceptance angle but scans linearly as a function of time. In both cases, the end result is that all points in the object have been observed from all possible angles. Although detailed calculations show that there are some differences between the two approaches, these differences are of secondary importance. The important issue for the clinician is whether it is better to collect the information from all the slices at the same time such that a volume of equal resolution in all three dimensions is available for reslicing in any direction (i.e., camera-based system) or whether it is more advantageous to be able to collect individual slices quickly and repeat the operation to obtain multiple slices (i.e., multicrystal scanner). With the latter method, if the patient moves, only the last scan has to be repeated rather than the entire procedure.

Positron Emission Tomographic Imaging

Overview. Positron emission tomographic (PET) imaging has been used as an important research tool and is now rapidly gaining acceptance as a clinical tool as well. This is largely due to the fact that there are important instrumentation and pharmaceutical characteristics that give PET imaging unique capabilities.

For some time now, the Anger scintillation camera has been the standard imaging device in nuclear medicine. Few significant improvements can be foreseen because system performance is limited by the collimator, which necessitates a trade-off between spatial resolution and sensitivity. Thus, further improvements in spatial resolution can be gained only by a sacrifice in sensitivity not acceptable with present-day radioisotopes. The severe restriction imposed by the collimator is illustrated by the fact that only 1 or 2 of the 10,000 gamma rays emitted from the body actually reach the detector. Furthermore, because system resolution is largely limited by the collimator, further improvements in intrinsic resolution would yield a negligible gain in overall image quality. With PET imaging, however, coincidence detection gives higher spatial resolution and higher sensitivity because a collimator is not necessary to localize the event, and little shielding is needed to reduce scattered radiation. The spatial resolution of PET scanners has been reduced dramatically during the past 10 years, from 15–20 mm FWHM in early scanners to better than 5 mm FWHM in present-day state-of-the-art scanners. Moreover, this gain in resolution has not been accompanied by a loss of sensitivity; rather, most present PET scanners image a minimum of seven transverse slices simultaneously with an in-plane sensitivity that is several hundred times higher than that of a gamma camera.

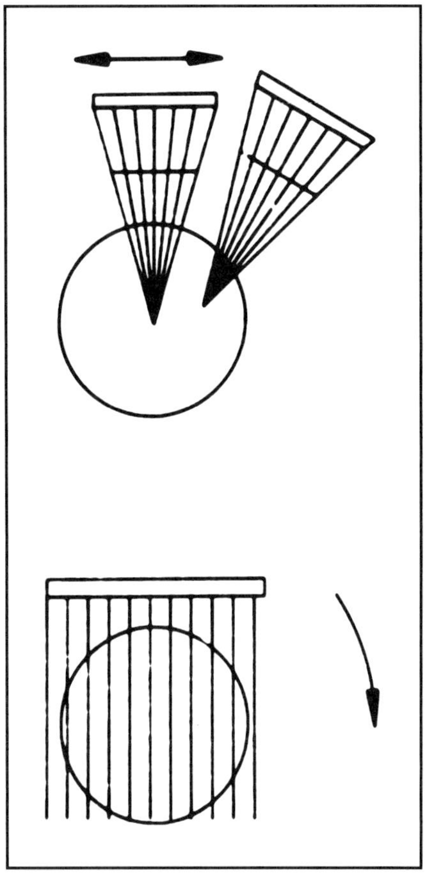

Figure 7 Successful emission computed tomographic imaging requires that all points be observed from all angles. This can be achieved by observing many angles simultaneously and then scanning linearly (top) or by sampling many linear points simultaneously and then scanning in the angular direction (bottom).

Positron emission tomographic imaging combines the advantages of high-resolution, high-sensitivity imaging with a wide range of unique radiopharmaceuticals that permit the study of neurological disease and myocardial function. The most interesting positron-emitting radionuclides are oxygen-15, carbon-11, nitrogen-13, and fluorine-18, with half-lives of 2, 10, 20, and 110 min, respectively. These nuclides, with the possible exception of fluorine-18, require an on-site cyclotron, and it was not until recently that compact cyclotrons became available for clinical use.

High-Resolution Scanners. One of the main attractions of PET imaging over single-photon gamma-ray imaging is the basic localization mechanism. A positron emitted from a radioactive substance will travel a short distance, combine with an electron, and annihilate. The range of the positron, which is proportional to its initial energy, limits the ultimate resolution of PET systems. The resulting energy is carried by two photons with an energy of 511 keV each that travel in nearly opposite directions. Simultaneous detection of two photons of this energy thus signals the decay of a positron anywhere along the line connecting the two points of detection. Because localization is achieved by coincidence detection and not by mechanical collimation of the photons, positron imaging can combine high spatial resolution with high detection efficiency because of the large solid angle for detecting pairs of annihilation photons.

Improvement in spatial resolution has typically been achieved by using a larger number of progressively smaller bismuth germanate (BGO) scintillation crystals. For example, the PET III scanner, one of the earliest systems, used 48

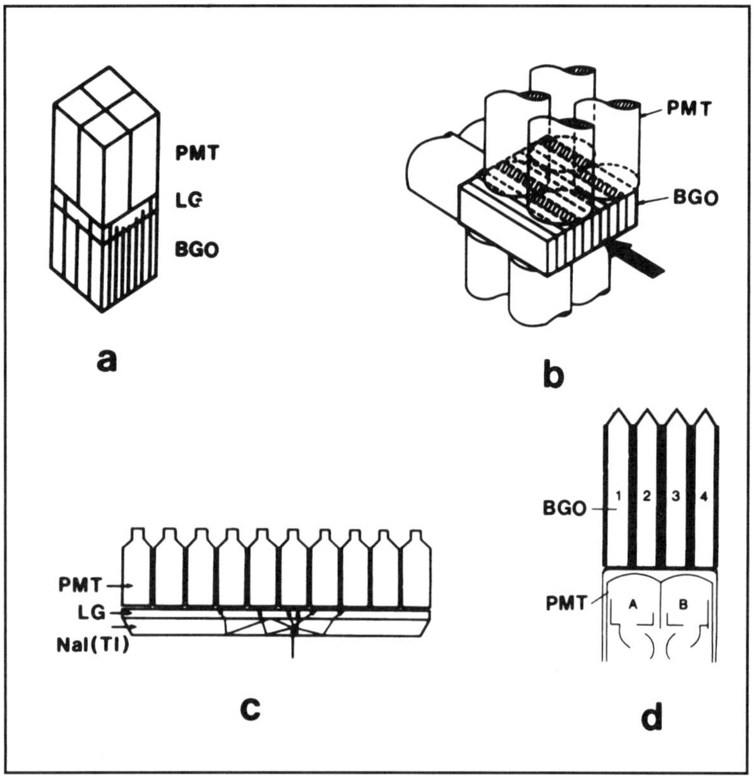

Figure 8 Numerous encoding schemes have been implemented to reduce detector complexity in positron emission tomographic scanners. Four representative methods, developed by (A) Computer Technology and Imaging (CTI), (B) Donner Laboratory, (C) University of Pennsylvania, and (D) Montreal Neurological Institute are shown. PMT = photomultiplier tube; LG = light guide; NaI(Tl) = sodium iodide crystal doped with thallium; BGO = bismuth germanate.

scintillation crystals; the Donner ring, the first high-resolution whole-body single-slice system, used 280 crystals arranged in a single ring; an ECAT III scanner used 512 crystals per ring; and the new PCR II being built by Brownell et al. uses more than 10,000 crystals in the complete system. To prevent the complexity and cost of the system from escalating as the number of crystals increases, more and more investigators are turning to encoding schemes that require fewer PMTs to yield a larger number of resolution elements. Several of these coding schemes are shown in Figure 8. A detailed discussion of the various encoding schemes is well beyond the scope of this syllabus; suffice it to say that the trend in positron scanners is toward systems with more resolution elements and fewer PMTs.

Effect of Resolution Improvement. Organs such as the brain and heart are high-contrast objects, and in the brain in particular, the smallest structure that one would visualize is significantly smaller than even the best resolution being contemplated in PET imaging. This accounts for the tremendous effort being made by several groups to improve the spatial resolution of these systems, and indeed, there has been great improvement in the quality of clinical images. The point is often made that high-quality ECT images need a very high count density and, as illustrated in Figure 9, image quality does in fact continue to improve as the count density increases. However, an equally significant improvement in image quality can be obtained by even a relatively modest improvement in spatial resolution (see Fig. 9). This argument applies mainly to high-contrast images encountered in ECT imaging rather than to low-contrast images typical in planar imaging.

As in SPECT imaging, the collected data must be corrected for various imperfections to yield quantitatively accurate three-dimensional representations of the radiopharmaceutical distribution. These corrections include subtraction of random coincidences and scatter background, correction for attenuation, and normalization to compensate for detector nonuniformity.

As spatial resolution improves in the transverse direction, it is also desirable to improve axial resolution. Whereas transverse resolution can be improved through the use of smaller crystals without a significant loss in sensitivity, axial resolution improvement leads to a proportional loss in sensitivity so long as only coincidences within a ring and between directly adjacent rings of detectors are accepted. This loss of sensitivity is avoided in volume-imaging PET scanners, which use a large axial acceptance angle while preserving good axial spatial resolution and axial sampling, which is approximately twice the spatial resolution (2-mm axial sampling, 5–6-mm axial resolution). This allows reslicing of the data into sagittal, coronal, and oblique sections without loss of image quality. The large axial acceptance angle leads to some loss in spatial resolution at a large radius unless a three-dimensional reconstruction algorithm is used.

Time-of-Flight Systems. In conventional PET imaging, two annihilation photons are detected in coincidence, defining a line through the target, the end points of which are given by the location of the detectors. The origin of the two photons (i.e., the point of annihilation of the positron) can be anywhere along that line when the coincidence resolving time is long (20 nsec) relative to the time it takes for the photons to traverse the distance between detectors. In time-of-flight (TOF)–assisted PET systems, the time difference between the arrival times of the two annihilation photons at the opposing detectors is measured to obtain additional information about the site of the positron annihilation within the object. The time difference between the arrival of the two photons is less than 1 nsec, and very good coincidence-resolving times (less than 300 psec) must therefore be achieved to gain meaningful additional information. Good timing information can be achieved only through careful choices with respect to scintillation crystals and PMTs. The main advantage of TOF PET imaging is an improvement in the signal-to-noise ratio through reduction in noise, but the technique also results in instruments with high count rate capability and good rejection of random coincidences, making TOF PET systems particularly useful for fast dynamic studies. However, in the process of optimizing these PET scanners for high count rate first-pass studies, some spatial resolution is typically sacrificed, making TOF systems inferior for most brain studies where count rate capability is less important than spatial resolution.

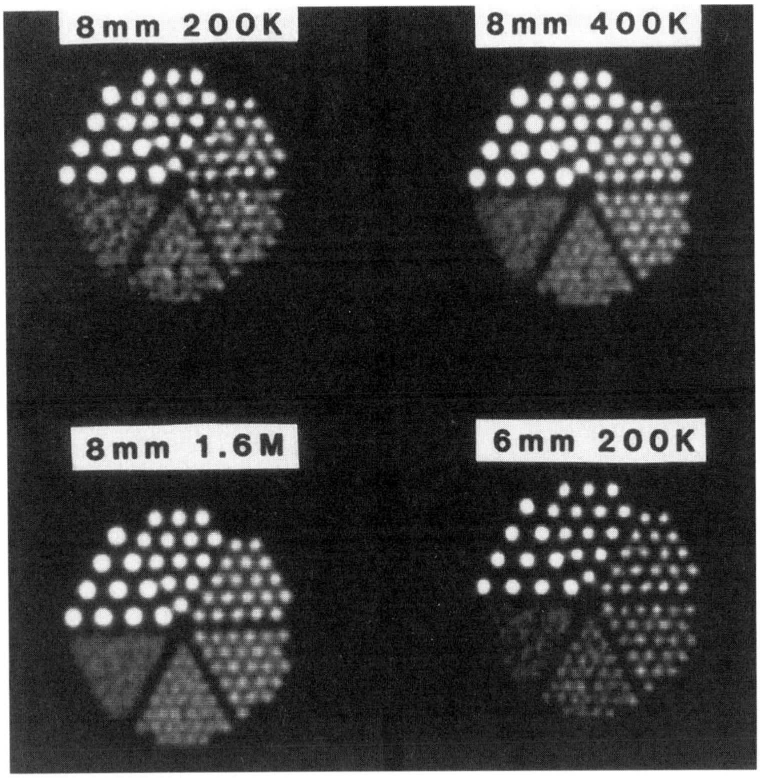

Figure 9 Image quality can be improved by acquiring more counts at a given spatial resolution or by improving the spatial resolution of the imaging instrument.

Summary

Most SPECT imaging is currently being performed with rotating Anger scintillation cameras. These are being enhanced with fan-beam and cone-beam collimators that increase sensitivity or spatial resolution, or both, depending on their design. Dedicated SPECT scanners are becoming available; in the most promising approach, the detectors are stationary, and only the collimator assembly rotates. However, these must be specifically designed for either brain or body imaging, whereas rotating Anger systems can be used equally well for both.

Aside from offering unique radiopharmaceutical tracers, PET imaging allows the use of imaging instruments that have significantly superior spatial resolution and sensitivity compared to SPECT imaging instruments. This performance is achieved by eliminating the need for mechanical collimation but results in more complex and therefore more costly devices.

NUCLEAR MEDICINE COMPUTERS

Parts of the Computer

A computer system used in a nuclear medicine laboratory consists of individual subsystems that together perform acquisition and analysis functions. Many of the components are common to almost all computer systems, whereas others are specialized. The parts that are found in all computers are the central processing unit (CPU), the memory, the disk drives, and the input/output devices. Other components that may be present are magnetic tape, data acquisition systems, and displays.

Central Processing Unit. Mathematical operations are performed by the CPU, which is designed to execute standard mathematical functions, such as addition, subtraction, multiplication, and division. As part of its processing capabilities, the CPU is able to make logical choices based on a comparison of two units of information. The CPU also has the ability to address memory and to decode instructions stored in memory, which it uses to determine how to process data.

Memory. Random access memory (RAM) is high-speed electronic storage for data and instructions. Memory is directly accessible to the CPU by a unique address and can be written into, as well as read from, as required by each operation of the CPU. Nuclear medicine computers can have many million storage locations, or bytes, of RAM. Sometimes the memory is divided into program memory and image memory, which are addressed separately. The programs that control the operations of the computer are stored in program memory, closely associated with the CPU. Image memory comprises a large array of storage locations that are used to collect and process nuclear medicine images.

Specialized RAM, called cache memory, is available on most recently designed small computers and greatly speeds up the operation of the system. Cache memory stores parts of programs or data that the CPU will access frequently. Because it is much faster than a disk or regular memory, cache memory can significantly improve the performance of the computer.

Magnetic and Optical Disk Drives. A computer disk system is composed of one or more platters of magnetic material bonded to a hard substrate and turned at high speed by a motor. Over the surfaces of the disk are suspended magnetic heads that enable the system to read and write data. The heads can be positioned directly over any part of the surface without touching it, making the magnetic disk system a random access device, as shown in Figure 10. Magnetic disks come in many sizes and designs (Tables 3–5), some of which permit the disks to be removed from the drive. They can range from single-platter systems, which store a few hundred megabytes of data, to high-capacity multiplatter systems with many heads that can store nearly 18 gigabytes (18 billion bytes). The data stored on magnetic disks will be information that cannot fit into RAM. Because of the storage capacity of a disk in relation to the cost, a disk provides cheaper storage of data than electronic memory.

Another type of disk, called the floppy diskette, uses a flexible, or "floppy," storage medium that cannot store as much information as a conventional disk drive. The floppy disk drive is relatively simple, and the diskette itself is inexpensive and removable, making it ideal for storing a few images at a time from an individual patient.

A recent technology, optical disk storage, is based on writing and reading information on a special platter by the use of lasers. The optical disk system has a major advantage over the conventional magnetic disk system in that the storage density of the device is very large. Storage of 1–2 gigabytes on each side of a removable 5¼ inch platter is typical, making the optical disk ideal for archiving large amounts of data that may need to be retrieved from time to time. Projections are that these devices will be able to store 100 gigabytes on a side. By designing a system that is like a jukebox with many platters, storage systems containing 1,000 gigabytes or more are possible. Coupled with an expected lifetime of 10–30 years, optical disks offer an ideal long-term storage capability for images.

Magnetic Tape. It is usually impractical to keep data that have been processed on disks for months or years because of the expense of the disk storage systems. The traditional long-term archival storage medium is reel-to-reel magnetic tape, which can store as much as 180 megabytes on a reel. Tape also is available in cassettes and cartridges that are similar to home audio and videotape cassettes. Modern designs of tape cassette and cartridge systems enable them to store as much as 8 to 18 billion bytes of information. The very high storage capacities are a result of newer ways of writing data on the tape than those used for conventional reel-to-reel systems.

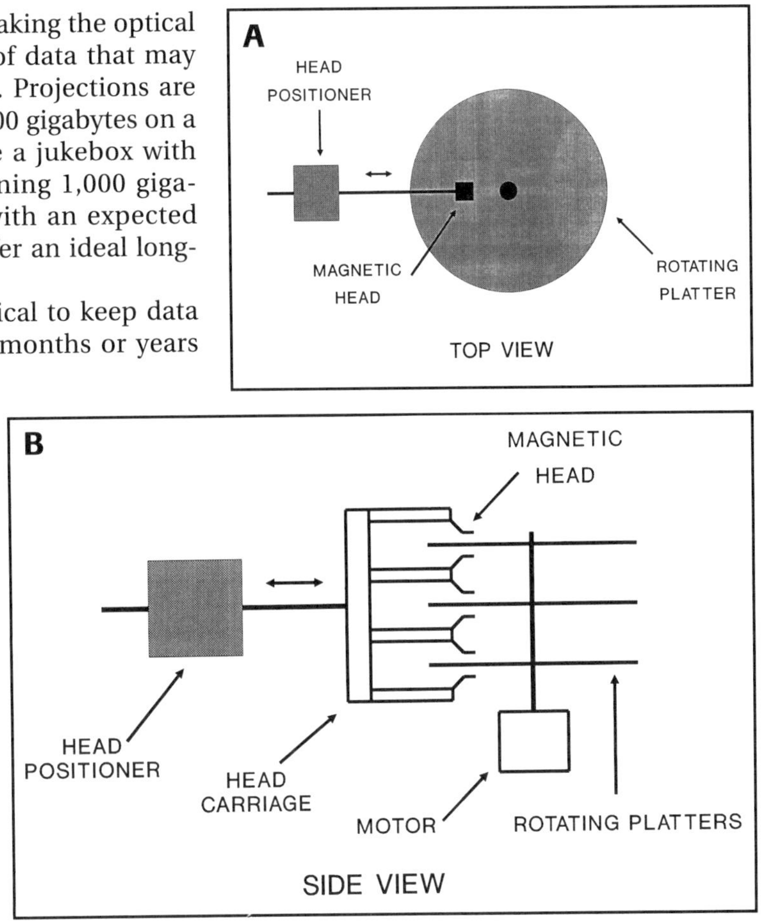

Figure 10 (A) Disk drives have a read/write head fixed on a movable arm so that the head can be positioned over any part of the disk. (B) Many disk systems have several platters, each accessed by its own head.

Analog-to-Digital Converters. An analog-to-digital converter (ADC) is an electronic circuit that is used to convert analog (continuously varying) signals to digital form so that the computer system can process them (Fig. 11). The two important signals that must be converted in a scintillation camera are the x- and y-coordinate signals. The Z pulse, derived from the pulse height analyzers, is used by the computer to activate a pair of ADCs to digitize these signals. An ADC can be designed in a number of ways, depending on the needs of the system, the accuracy equired, the speed of conversion, and the necessary resolution. Errors can be introduced during the conversion process and can include accuracy errors, gain shifts, differential nonlinearity, and integral nonlinearity. Depending on the system design, should these errors occur, they can significantly affect image quality.

Analog-to-digital converters are available that digitize signals to 8, 10, or 12 bits of accuracy. As the conversion resolution increases, the time required for conversion also increases. Because modern cameras can produce count rates in excess of 200,000 cps, an ADC must be able to convert the analog camera signals to digital form very rapidly to avoid significant count loss. Conversion times of 1.5 μsec or better are required. Most nuclear medicine computer systems are designed to be connected to as many as four cameras at once. However, some machines have a single pair of ADCs, so that data can only be collected from one camera at a time. Other systems can perform simultaneous acquisitions because they either have more than one pair of ADCs or use multiplexers and high-speed ADCs to process signals from several cameras. The advantage of multiple simultaneous acquisitions is that a single computer serves more than

Table 3
STORAGE CAPACITY FOR MAGNETIC DISKS

Type	Size (in.)	Storage (megabytes)
Floppy diskette	3½	1.44–2.88
	5¼	1.2
Single hard disk (removable)	5¼	100–1000
Multplatter hard disk (nonremovable)	3½	200–4300
	5¼	2000–18000
	5¼	20–500
	8	600
	14	1,200

Note sizes tend to double every 10-12 months

Table 4
STORAGE CAPACITY OF TAPE SYSTEMS

Density	Length (feet)	Storage (megabytes)
1,600 BPI reel-to-reel	600	11.5
	1,200	23
	2,400	46
6,250 BPI reel-to-reel	600	45
	1,200	90
	2,400	180
Regular cartridge	450	40–60
Video cartridge	750	1,200

BPI = bits per inch

Table 5
STORAGE CAPACITY OF OPTICAL DISKS

Type	Size (in.)	Storage (megabytes)
Single side	5¼	500
	12	1,000
Dual side	12	2,000

one camera, so that expensive components do not have to be duplicated. However, the computer's software must support multiple acquisition tasks, making it more complex.

Display Systems. Nuclear medicine computers include a video display, where the physician reviews the results of a study. Available displays are 256 × 256 or 512 × 512 picture element (pixel) resolution, although some review workstations intended for use in a picture network have 1,024 × 1,024 capability. The display system is usually capable of showing 256 levels of gray in each pixel and can be equipped with overlay planes for text and graphic overlay of images.

Image information that is acquired at low spatial resolutions is often displayed as an interpolated image so that it fills more of the screen. An image acquired with a scintillation camera in a 64 × 64 matrix might be interpolated up to 256 × 256 pixels on the display screen. Interpolation is a mathematical process in which values of pixels in a high-resolution image are found by calculating a linear average value between the pixels in a low-resolution image. The original pixel values and the newly calculated interpolated values are placed in a larger image matrix. The interpolation process does not increase the spatial resolution of the interpolated images but does remove some of the "blocky" character that is sometimes seen when low-resolution images are enlarged without interpolation.

A color display system used to be an option on nuclear medicine computers, but so many analysis programs use color that it is now standard equipment. The color that is displayed is arbitrarily assigned to the value in each pixel through lookup tables and can be used to highlight subtle differences between numbers of counts that might otherwise be difficult to detect on a gray-scale display. The computer can change the appearance of a color image by changing the way counts are assigned to colors. This permits the physician to develop assignment tables for particular purposes, especially for representing quantitative information.

Display Interaction. Interaction with information displayed on the image screen is accomplished either by entering commands into the computer from the keyboard or by using some type of dynamic device (Fig. 12) to position a visible cursor at desired points on the displayed image. Of five devices used with medical imaging computer systems, the most popular is the joystick. It is connected to the display electronics so that movement of the joystick produces a corresponding movement of the cursor on the screen. The base of the device remains stationary while the arm is pointed in the direction that the cursor should move. Other devices used for the same function are the trackball and mouse, which provide the user with more precise positioning of the cursor than the joystick. A light pen or digitizing tablet can also be used.

Computer Software

Operating Systems. A computer program is an implementation of an algorithm, which is simply a recipe for doing something useful in a step-by-step manner. A program designed for a particular application contains the commands that the computer can execute to perform a specified function.

Although specialized programs are used for nuclear medicine acquisition and analysis, the control of the computer system is based on a collection of programs called the operating system. These tools, provided by the manufacturer of the computer, permit a user's program to interact with the various parts of the computer system. In effect, the operating system provides an environment for other programs, called application programs, to function. The operating system has several basic capabilities that enable the computer user to perform useful functions. It provides the means for input and output of information to the user; it provides communication with the hardware devices that are part of the computer; and it provides important housekeeping functions, such as recording where information is stored, how much room is occupied by the information, and whether the device storing the information is available for use. As the computer system becomes more elaborate, the operating system takes on additional functions related to scheduling when events occur and managing information flow through the system. These functions are not apparent to the users, but they are essential to the operation of the system.

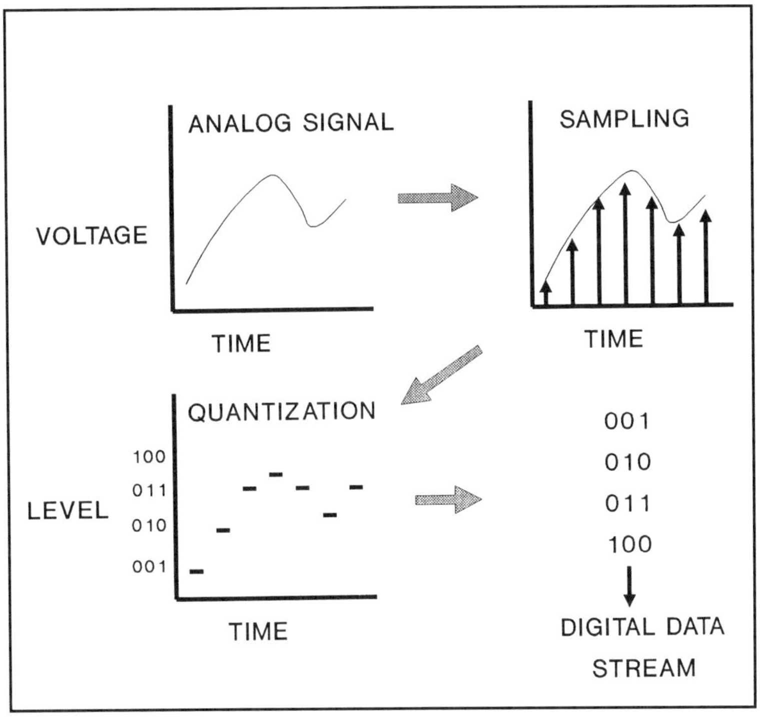

Figure 11 Analog-to-digital converters incorporate electronic circuits that sample, quantize, and assign digital values to continuously varying signals from a scintillation camera.

Types of Operating Systems. For many years, small nuclear medicine computers have used a single-user operating system. In this design one user has command of the entire computer. It performs one task at a time according to the commands received. The operating system does not need to be complex and is appropriate for small nuclear medicine departments where acquisition and processing operations do not have to occur at the same time.

An enhancement of this approach is the foreground–background operating system, which gives priority of the computer to a real-time data collection operation running in the foreground, such as event detection from a gamma camera. An analysis program, running in the background, is suspended until the real-time event has been properly processed. Then the computer lets the background program function again, toggling rapidly between the two tasks to give the appearance of doing two things at once.

As users have demanded higher performance from their nuclear medicine computers and the cost of such performance has gone down, there has been an increased use of multitasking operating systems. This type of operating system permits several time-critical or real-time operations to run by assigning a priority to each task, based on how often the operation must be serviced, as de-

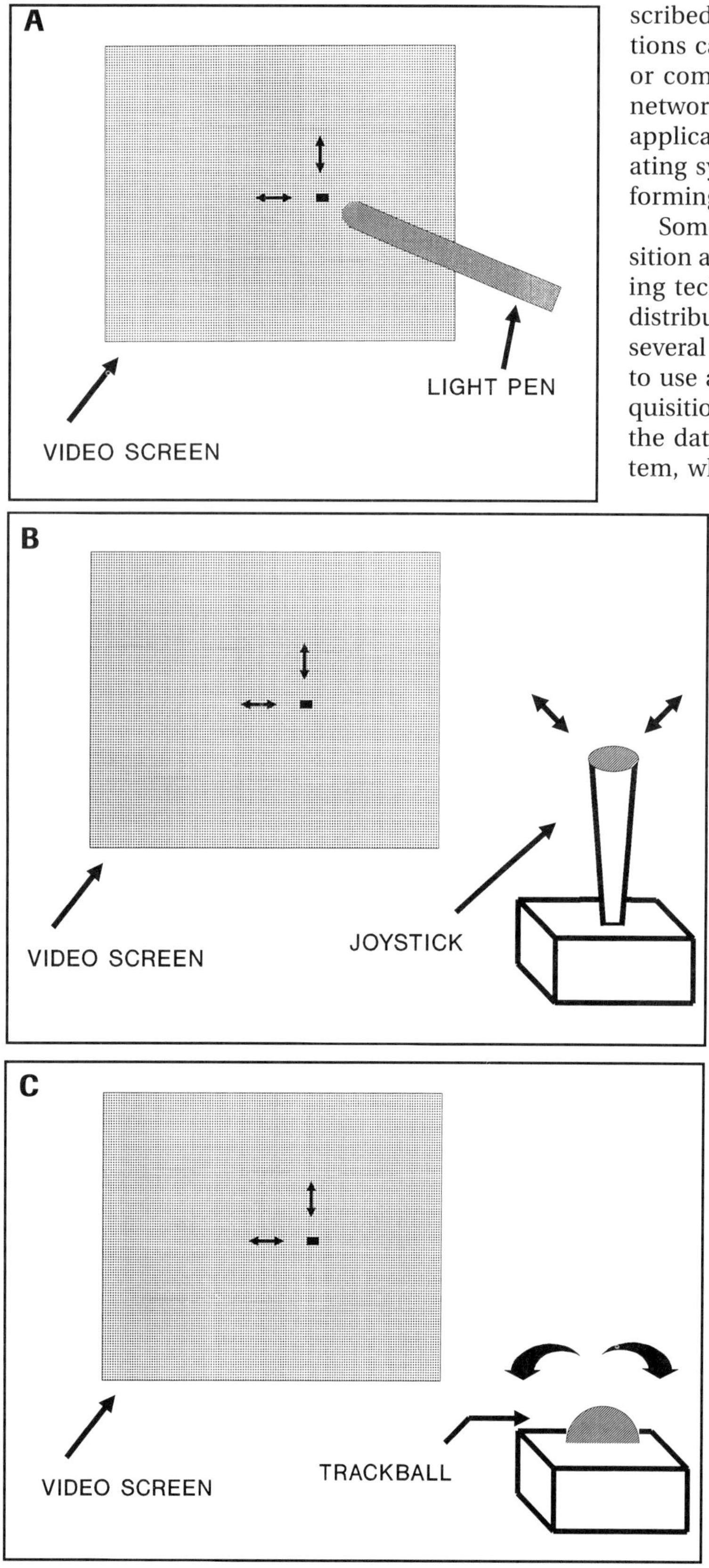

scribed in Figure 13. Several background functions can occur as well, such as image analysis or communication with other computers on a network. If the computer is fast enough and the applications are properly matched to the operating system, the computer appears to be performing several different functions at once.

Some new designs of nuclear medicine acquisition and processing systems use multiprocessing techniques in which the operating system distributes the load on the computer system over several separate CPUs. The usual arrangement is to use a CPU with its own memory for data acquisition while the master or main CPU operates the data analysis programs. The operating system, which is multitasking, supports the separate processors, ensuring that each has the proper programs in place for the function that is being performed. The advantage to this design is that the system can offer very high performance, both for data acquisition and analysis.

Utility Software. All operating systems have certain programs performing similar types of mundane but necessary functions needed in day-to-day use of the computer, no matter what the design. These programs are known as system utilities. They provide the user with the capability to determine information about available resources, print the contents of disk storage areas, copy information from one place to another, delete old information, and compress unused space on disk drives. Additionally, utility programs are usually provided to perform special operations related to nuclear medicine acquisition and analysis.

Figure 12 Interactive cursor control devices assist the user in selecting parts of an image on the screen. (A) The light pen is held in the hand against the screen. The cursor is positioned on the screen wherever the pen is located. (B) The joystick causes the cursor to be moved on the screen to correspond to the position of the joystick arm. (C) The trackball positions the cursor by rolling the ball in the direction in which the cursor must be moved. The trackball provides more accurate positioning than the light pen or joystick.

Networks. The trend in nuclear medicine departments is to integrate many of the functions previously accommodated by several independent computers into a network. A network is a collection of computers that are linked to each other by some form of high-speed communication system, enabling movement of information from one machine to another for specialized processing or review. The computers connected to the network can include those that are capable of supporting data acquisition and processing independent of the network. Other machines may be collection-only or analyze-only computers, called workstations, that depend on a larger, faster computer on the network to provide many of the resources that the other machines lack, especially large amounts of data storage. This "server" performs complex processing and archiving operations for the other smaller computers by sharing data over the network. In some large nuclear medicine departments, a number of review workstations are connected to the server. In this arrangement, images are collected from acquisition workstations, sent by the network to the server, then transmitted to any of the review workstations at the request of physicians. Archiving of these data is performed at the server, so that the entire network becomes a picture-archiving system (PACS). Such a system can be connected to a larger radiology PACS so that all picture information for a particular patient can be made available to the physician.

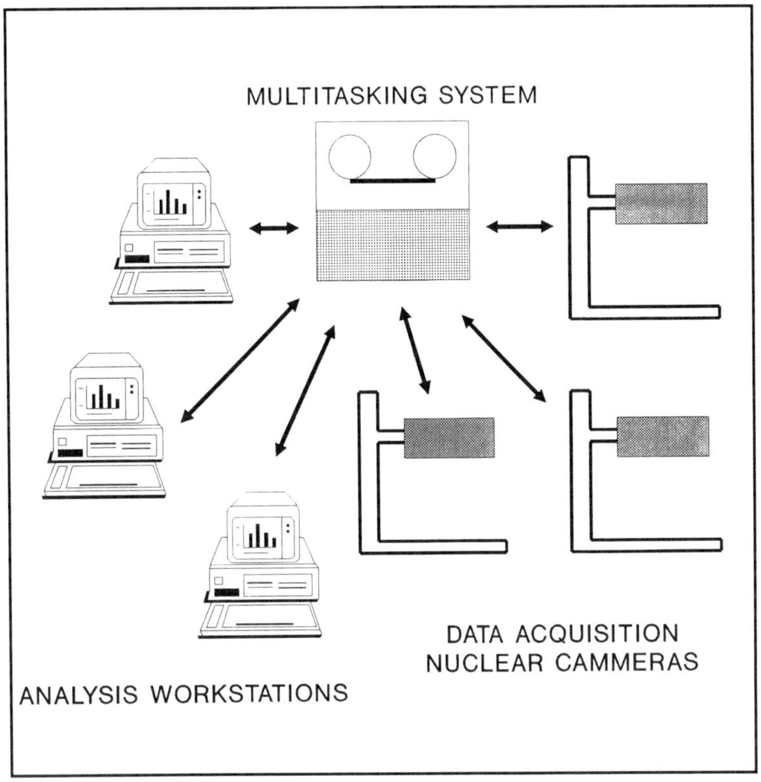

Figure 13 A multitasking operating system permits several real-time data collection operations to occur at the same time as several analysis operations that are not real time.

Computer Languages. Programs are written in a structured form called a computer language that has a syntax and vocabulary, as does any written language. A computer language is designed to permit the human programmer to formulate algorithms into a program relatively easily and efficiently. The program is processed by another program, a language translator, which produces a sequence of binary numbers that the CPU can interpret as instructions and data.

There are three "classes" of computer languages: assembly languages, interpreted languages, and compiled languages. *Assembly languages* are very highly specific to a particular computer design and consist of short, often cryptic mnemonics that refer to specific functions that a CPU can perform. An assembly language program is compact, usually very efficient, and controls the detailed operation of the computer. Assembly language programs are used as the components of an operating system or for data collection where speed and efficiency are important.

Interpreted languages are much more removed from the terse and difficult form of assembly language. Interpreters permit the programmer to create programs using a syntax and vocabulary that are much more like English than assembly language. An interpreter converts lines of a program into executable statements and executes each one as it is converted every time the program is run. This has the advantage that errors are immediately apparent to the user but may not be very efficient in the way that the interpreter must use the resources of the computer. The most common interpreted language, BASIC, has been used in nuclear medicine for a variety of processing operations, especially in those situations where the programming requirements are fairly routine and speed is not very important.

Compilers are complex language translation programs that convert a program in a source language to a machine-usable form, usually with an intermediate step. There is no instant execution of each line of the program as it is being converted. However, the compilation process only has to be done once. Then, each time the program must be run, it executes very rapidly because it has already been converted to a usable form. FORTRAN, C, and Pascal are compiled languages used for programming in nuclear medicine.

NUCLEAR MEDICINE ACQUISITION SOFTWARE

The User Interface

The nuclear medicine software presents itself to the user in one of three ways. The first is a menu-based system where the user selects options from a list displayed on the screen. Often the choice is made by typing its number or by pushing a special function key on the keyboard to advance to the selected operation. Sometimes it is necessary to traverse several such menus to get to the desired function.

A variation on the menu-based system involves the use of menus that are activated by a mouse or trackball pointing device. In this type of system, the menus appear in "windows" over parts of the screen. The computer system instantaneously presents a menu at the selection of a function with the cursor. The advantage of this technique is that it retains the ease of use of a conventional menu system but is very fast because of the mouse-controlled cursor and the ability of the system to display several menus that overlap each other.

The third method of interacting with the nuclear medicine software uses few or no menus to perform operations. Instead, the user must enter a command at a prompt. The user must be familiar with the available commands and formats, which usually requires a substantial period of training before proficiency is achieved. The user of the command-driven system typically has the option of combining a number of commands into a file, often called a "macro," that can be invoked by a single command.

Static Image Acquisition Programs

A static image is an image collected directly into the computer's memory, under the control of a static acquisition program. Static images are formed by incrementing by one each memory location corresponding to an xy position in the camera. The image is built up point by point until either the operator stops the collection, or a preset number of counts (Z pulses) is reached, or the image starts to overflow, or a specified collection duration is achieved. When acquisition stops, the image is stored on disk for later review.

The program usually permits the user to specify the matrix size that the image will have in pixels, typically 64×64, 128×128, or 256×256. The program may also permit the user to specify how many bits, representing the maximum number of counts, will be used for each pixel. Eight bits can represent up to 255 counts, whereas 16 bits represent 65,535 counts. Ordinarily, it is preferable to use 16-bit collections so that some of the pixels in the static image do not overflow by exceeding 255. When overflow occurs during an 8-bit acquisition, some software designs set the next value after 255 to zero. Other software monitors the values in each pixel, halting the collection at overflow.

Dynamic Acquisition Programs

A dynamic acquisition program permits the computer system to collect data over time in order to follow the temporal progression of a physiological process. The computer system acquires a sequence of static images automatically, allowing each static image to build for a set length of time, then begins accumulating the next image in the sequence. If the computer has enough RAM, the software can store all the images in memory. On completion of the entire study, the images are written to disk. If there is not enough RAM to store the images, the program can be designed to use a method called double buffering, where two collection locations are allocated in memory. While one location is being filled by the program, the other is written to disk. The program toggles between the two until the collection is complete. With this technique the size of the disk is the limit to the number of images that can be collected.

Most systems permit different dynamic collection protocols. Multiple-phase dynamic acquisitions, in which the time of the collection of frames changes under control of the acquisition programs, can be used to monitor a physiological process that begins rapidly and then slows down. This capability makes it possible to match the acquisition to the dynamic needs of the situation.

Gated Studies

A gated study is most often used to collect images for evaluation of cardiac variables. Gated collections can be performed as a specialized dynamic study or in an unformatted mode, called list mode acquisition. A gated collection uses the timing signal from detection of the QRS complex of the electrocardiogram to control the acquisition of data into several frames that are defined in the computer's memory. When the gated collection is initialized, the user tells the program how many frames to allocate at a particular matrix size and how many bits to allocate for each pixel, as in static collections. The user also tells the program the stopping criterion for the acquisition. The stopping criterion can be total number of counts, total elapsed time, total number of cardiac cycles accepted, occurrence of an overflow, or a manual termination.

The collection program detects the time interval between successive R waves (the RR interval) and calculates the amount of time that each frame should receive by dividing the RR interval time by the number of frames selected for the collection. As the acquisition begins, the first R wave is detected, and the program begins to store the incoming data into the first frame. When the calculated time for the frame is reached, data are stored in the next frame in succession. This process continues through all the frames spaced over the RR interval. At the beginning of the second detected R wave, the process begins again by storing counts in the first frame. Over time, a sequence of images representing different phases of the cardiac cycle is built up in memory. When the defined stopping criterion is reached, the images are stored on disk for later analysis.

A potential problem with this scheme arises because of irregular heart rates and bad beats that occur with some patients. Because the computer has no way of knowing whether an RR interval is too long or too short until the interval is over, it cannot reject the data from the bad beat. What is usually done is to reject data from the next RR interval, although this procedure may not be appropriate for many types of arrhythmias. It is possible with fast computers and a large amount of RAM to create an intermediate frame buffer (storage area) before summing beats into each frame. With this approach, data from a bad beat can be rejected before being summed into the images in memory. Gated list mode acquisition to disk can also be used so that bad beats can be properly rejected when the data are assembled into images after collection.

List Mode Acquisition

List mode acquisition and gated list mode acquisition are nonframe types of acquisitions in which a list of digitized x and y coordinates are recorded on disk along with timing information for later formatting into images. List mode acquisitions ordinarily are used when high count rates are expected or when patients with irregular heart rates must be imaged. Double buffering or other techniques ensure that high count rates can be accommodated by the system.

A gated list mode study is essentially the same as regular list mode acquisition, except that both timing information and the time of an R-wave trigger pulse are stored. The resulting list on disk contains all the necessary information to construct sequences of gated images, a process called reframing. Because the images are created after the collection, bad beats and their associated data can be rejected from the image set during the reframing operation.

In list mode acquisition, the data can be reframed into different array sizes with different times per frame. Images can be produced in which the RR interval is divided into equal time intervals or into a fixed number of intervals. Reframing methods have been demonstrated that compensate for drop-off of count rates in late diastole. These techniques involve "reverse framing" from the next detected R-wave pulse. When combined with conventional forward framing, a composite series is created in which both diastole and systole are properly presented.

Single-Photon Emission Computed Tomographic Systems Data Acquisition

The nuclear medicine computer system with options for SPECT imaging can interact with the SPECT camera in two ways. The computer can control the motion of the camera directly through a digital link to the positioning system, or it can receive position information from the camera, which is under the control of its own electronics. The latter might be called a slave mode because the computer follows the data acquisition but is not in control of it. Conventional camera signals are provided to the computer system through the camera interface.

During SPECT acquisitions, the computer system will automatically acquire a series of images, usually 64 for every 180° rotation of the camera, assuming filtered backprojection reconstruction. The computer or the camera's electronics causes the camera to rotate around a patient who is positioned at the center of rotation. Depending on the acquisition programs, the camera either stops at each point, collects data as a planar image, then steps to the next point to collect the next planar images or scans continuously, very slowly, around the patient. With the step-and-shoot acquisition method, planar images are usually available as "monitor" images during acquisition. The processing programs reformat the images into projections that are used in the reconstruction process.

NUCLEAR MEDICINE PROCESSING SOFTWARE

There are many different types of programs that have been written to analyze data acquired during a nuclear medicine procedure. In general, these programs take an image or set of images and permit the user to interact with the image data to yield quantitative functional information in a specific area of the image. Some of the programs use complex processing methods that transform the raw images into specialized images showing dynamic characteristics of the organ of interest. These methods are discussed in detail in published reports. Most types of analysis use the collected images from which data are selected on a regional basis and used to form curves representing changes in activity with time. These more widely applicable methods are discussed here.

Image Manipulation

Many types of image manipulation are used in preparing nuclear medicine data for viewing and quantitative processing. One of the simplest is called windowing, or thresholding, a procedure that lets the user match the range of collected data to the capabilities of the display system. The concept behind windowing is that the data, in counts per pixel, that must be displayed may exceed the range of the display to accommodate them. Most displays show 256 gray-scale levels or colors, and data may have count values as high as 65,535. An upper and lower threshold value is specified that creates a window of gray levels into the pixel values in the image. Every pixel value less than the specified lower threshold appears to be black on the screen, whereas every value above the upper threshold appears to be white. Those values in between are mapped to the 256-level range of the display. If the window is wider than 256 levels, then some loss of gray resolution will occur; if the window is less than 256 levels wide, then some contouring or sudden transition from one visible gray level to the next may be noticeable. If a color table is in use, then the threshold procedure overlays the range of the color table. Threshold values can be changed at will by the user and do not alter the original data in any way.

Another type of image processing operation that is used is image filtering. Two-dimensional filters are used to smooth images to make them more viewable by removing or reducing noise and to enhance edges. An example is the five-point smoothing filter, which performs a moving average on each pixel in the image. The pixel to be smoothed is multiplied by a weighting function and summed with its four orthogonal neighbors, also multiplied by a weighting function, to yield the smoothed pixel value. This value then replaces the original pixel value.

Other types of two-dimensional filters can be implemented in the Fourier domain. This means that the image is processed by a two-dimensional fast Fourier transformation (FFT) program, which converts the spatial domain image into the frequency domain. The frequency domain values are an array of spatial frequencies that, taken together, describe the original image. By multiplying these frequency values by an appropriate filter function, various parts of the frequency array can be changed with respect to their contributions to the image. After this has been done, the frequency array is processed by an inverse FFT to produce the filtered image. It is much easier to design complex filters using FFT methods if the time required for the computation is of secondary importance.

Temporal filtering is another type of processing that is applied to multiple images, such as in a dynamic cardiac study. In a typical temporal smoothing operation, the value of a given pixel at a specific location in an image is multiplied by a weighting factor and summed with the corresponding pixel multiplied by a weighting factor in the immediately preceding and following images. The resulting value replaces the original pixel. The formulation is similar to the three-point smoothing operation used to filter curves. Corresponding pixels in a temporally related image set form time–activity curves. Thus, temporal filtering is a smoothing of all the time–activity curves that form the images. Sometimes the temporal filter can contain contributions from several images before and after the selected image. The smoothing that usually results is somewhat different from single-image filter functions because there is less loss of spatial resolution, but there is a reduction in noise. However, temporal information is also lost.

Regions of Interest

Regions of interest (ROIs) are parts of an image that are selected for purposes of analysis, usually by outlining the region on the image screen. A pointing device, such as a joystick, is used to move a visible cursor on the screen around the ROI. As the cursor moves, the ROI is surrounded by a trail of dots, indicating the boundary of the region. To complete the selection, the boundary must be closed. All the counts in all the pixels within the ROI are taken together for purposes of analysis.

The ROI can have an irregular shape or a geometric shape, such as a circle or rectangle. For geometric shapes, it is not necessary to outline the region. Usually, two opposite corners of a rectangle can be used to specify its boundaries. Likewise, the center and radius of a circle can be used by the ROI program to select a circular region on the image. The program creates the boundary for the ROI and places it on the screen. Many systems permit ROIs to be moved on the screen or changed in size. Often, more than one ROI will be used for a particular analysis protocol, separating information into different parts of the image.

Curve Processing

Time–activity curves are plotted representations of the behavior of detected activity within selected corresponding ROIs in a series of images collected over time (Fig. 14). One or more ROIs are chosen over parts of the first image in the temporally separated image set. The same ROI is used for each subsequent image in the series. From each ROI a number is derived related to some manipulation of the counts in the selected region. The number most often represents the total counts, the maximum or minimum of the counts, or the average count in the ROI. This number is obtained from the ROI in each image in the data set and is plotted on a scale of counts versus time. These curves might be used in analysis of the washout of activity from a kidney over time or the passage of labeled red cells through the left ventricle, among other possible uses.

Curves can be processed in many ways to enhance interpretation of the information. Processing can be fairly simple and includes addition, subtraction, multiplication, and division of the curve values by constants. Somewhat more com plex manipulations can include algebraic manipulation by corresponding points on a curve with the same time interval as the original. Points on a curve can be summed together to find values for a longer time interval than the original curve. The slope of part of the curve can be determined to show the rate of change of activity.

Noisy curves are those whose values change abruptly. These curves can be filtered using various one-dimensional smoothing operations. These filters can use the FFT but are more easily implemented for simple smoothing as a running weighted average. An example of a filter is the three-point moving average filter:

Nc = (W1)(C1) + (W2)(C) + (W3)(C2),

where Nc is the number of counts after filtering; W1, W2, and W3 are weighting factors, C1 is the number of counts at the previous point; C is the number of counts at the current point; and C2 is the number of counts at the next point; Nc replaces C after filtering. The weighting factors add together to equal 1, so that the overall image intensity is not altered.

Much more elaborate processing operations can be performed on time–activity curves. As an example, in first-pass studies of left-to-right shunts and in renograms, the bolus of radioactive tracer is injected as rapidly as possible into a vein. However, broadening of the time–activity curve during passage of the bolus through the vascular system occurs. Observation of the time–activity curve detected at the target organ shows a curve exhibiting the characteristics of both the target organ and the vascular system.

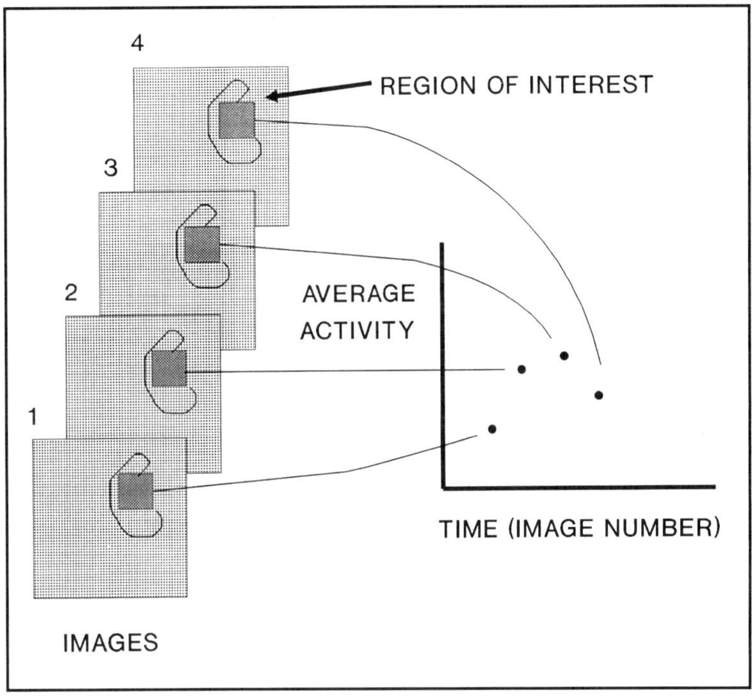

Figure 14 Time–activity curve produced from a region of interest (ROI) selected on the first image of a temporally related series of images or selected separately on each image of the series. The count values are then processed, often by averaging, and plotted as activity versus time, where each successive image represents advancing time.

For left-to-right shunts, the input time–activity curve from the vena cava can be measured, as can the output time–activity curve over the lungs. A mathematical process known as deconvolution permits the user to compute an approximation of an ideal time–activity curve that would result from instantaneous injection of contrast medium into the target. The relation is described mathematically by a convolution operation where the input function convolved with the actual response of the pulmonary system equals the observed output time–activity curve. By using deconvolutsion, the actual time–activity curve representing the response of the pulmonary system alone can be found from the observed curve.

Count Profiles

It is often of interest to be able to create a plot of number of counts per pixel verses pixel position in an image. Such a plot is called a count profile and is most often linear but can be circular or irregularly shaped. The purpose is to display the intensity seen in the image so that the relationships between different count levels along the profile can be appreciated more easily.

For linear count profiles, the user selects the extent of the plot by positioning the cursor at a starting position on an image. The cursor is then moved to another position, and a profile is produced for the straight line drawn between the two cursor positions. The plot usually appears at the bottom of the image screen as an overlay over the image. Some systems permit multiple linear profiles to be plotted simultaneously, making comparison between parts of an image easier.

Much more elaborate processing can be performed based on profile curve usage. A useful approach to cardiac processing can be found in quantitation or thallium perfusion SPECT images to determine the location and extent of myocardial ischemia. This approach is known as bull's eye analysis. In this method radial lines are placed on each short axis slice, usually at 6 degree increments from a central point, starting at the apex and proceeding to the base of the heart. For each slice a circumferential profile is produced from the intersection of each radial line with the peak detected activity. All of the circumferential profiles are plotted on a display with the apex in the center, moving towards the base. The intensity of the display at a point represents the magnitude of activity in a slice and the location of the point on the bull's eye indicates the slice location. Since the bull's eye plots are presented in a standard orientation from data acquired with a defined protocol, comparison can be made to a database of normal and abnormal studies, thereby asissting in the interpretation of the study.

Circumferential profiles are computed from collected left anterior oblique (LAO) image data plus two other images at somewhat different orientations. The user outlines the left and right ventricles with a rectangular ROI. The computer performs a background subtraction using a bilinear interpolation method and a nine-point moving average smooth of the selected region. The center of the left ventricle is then located manually. The computer proceeds to form radial lines from the center of the ventricle. In the Cedars-Sinai method, 60 radial segments with a 6° arc are produced, with the maximum radial distance specified by the operator. The computer next finds the pixels representing the maximum counts in each radial section. From these, the circumferential profile is computed. The user interacts with the program at this point to choose the left ventricular apex. The computer then plots the circumferential profile clockwise from 0° to 360°, with the apex at 90°. Normalization to the maximum in the profile is performed before plotting. From these plots the program proceeds to produce a comprehensive display showing the essential features of the thallium distribution in the form of three concentric rings for each projection: The innermost is the myocardial shape, the center the initial thallium distribution, and the outermost the washout of thallium. Discontinuities in the center or outer ring show abnormal distribution or washout, respectively, when compared to the values in the database of normal profiles. Extensive validation of the method at many institutions has been reported.

Single-Photon Emission Computed Tomographic Processing Programs

The nature of data acquisition in SPECT imaging requires that the software available for image reconstruction and processing be quite different and often more elaborate from that used in conventional nuclear medicine data processing. These requirements dictate that the computer system employ more powerful processing equipment than would be necessary in a routine imaging environment. Likewise, the programs required are more complex to write and often more complex to use.

Reconstruction of SPECT data is performed by using the method of filtered backprojection. In this reconstruction technique, the data from each input image provide projections of a collection of planes perpendicular to the input images through the patient. During the process of reconstruction, projection information from an individual input image is first modified mathematically in a process called filtering, then projected back across the transverse plane, and algebraically summed with projections from all the other raw images around the transverse plane.

The selection of the filter function used in filtered backprojection has been the subject of considerable investigation. In fact, most SPECT computer systems permit the user to select reconstructions using one of several different filters. In many cases, one particular filter may be preferred for liver reconstructions, whereas another might be used with gated heart studies. Among the types of filters available are the Hann, Hamming, Parzen, Ramp, and Butterworth filters. Butterworth filters can be specified by cutoff frequency and order, thereby allowing the user to change the behavior of the filter for a particular situation. A user-designed filter capability is usually included.

Because the display of reconstructed data is different from conventional two-dimensional data, SPECT software will include the capability to display the three-dimensional image set. The most important capability is to display all three orthogonal views of the organ of interest: sagittal, transverse, and coronal. Some display software will permit the user to see all orthogonal views on one screen with a line through each view that corresponds to the single slice that is also displayed. This arrangement is often interactive so that the user can move the slice line with a pointing device, displaying the corresponding slice. Zoom capability may be part of the display, as well as various cine display modes.

New display methods that permit the user to see the surfaces of an organ are of considerable interest. These methods use the transverse sectional images from a SPECT data set, which are reformatted and processed so that the appearance on the screen is a two-dimensional image representing the surface of a three-dimensional structure. If the computer system is fast enough, or the views have been previously selected and calculated, the organ can be rotated on the screen by displaying images in a movie loop. By varying the way that the data are processed, different surfaces can be presented or transparency added, permitting the observer to "look through" part of the organ to see a deep structure.

SYSTEM MANAGEMENT

Quality Assurance of Computer Equipment

Computer hardware is extremely reliable, but problems can occur that affect the ability of the computer to acquire, process, display, and archive image data. Some parts of the computer can even change their characteristics over time, altering the way they function.

The most likely parts of a nuclear medicine computer to change characteristics are the ADCs used to digitize the camera signals. Analog circuits are subject to drift and other instabilities, either because of design deficiencies or aging of components. Such changes associated with ADCs that are part of the camera interface can cause subtle alterations in the appearance of images. To detect these changes, quality assurance phantoms should be used on a regular basis. Analysis of these images will assist the user in determining the functional capability of the acquisition and analysis system and will indicate when recalibration is required. Other parts of the computer system, those that are purely "digital," tend to either work or not, so a problem is often obvious. However, under some circumstances, a component of the digital electronics may fail, resulting in either loss of information or (rarely) an incorrect calculation.

Software, especially new application programs, is often difficult to evaluate. In most facilities, software that is used clinically has been extensively evaluated and validated in that facility or is supplied by the manufacturer as validated at an independent laboratory. Software may contain errors that only appear under unusual conditions of data acquisition or processing. New or updated software, either written in-house or obtained from outside, must be validated by the users before being installed for routine clinical imaging.

Validation of software involves the use of either extensive data sets that when processed have known results, or, perhaps better, the use of side-by-side comparison of the processing software with a "gold standard" examination that provides the basis of comparison. Sometimes it becomes difficult to ensure that the software is providing the user with the information intended. It is therefore the user's obligation to question the results of any processing program and to look for unreasonable and inconsistent results in day-to-day use.

Archiving and Backup

Archiving usually refers to storing patient studies so that they can be retrieved and reviewed at a later date. Backup refers to storing extra copies of programs and the operating system so that the operation of the computer can be restored quickly if a problem occurs that damages the working copy of the software. Archiving will usually be performed daily or every few days, depending on the patient load on the computer system.

Ordinarily, the programs and operating system only need to be backed up when something changes, such as the addition of a new cardiac analysis program or an upgrade to a new revision of the operating system. The goal is to maintain an exact duplicate of the working software system so that it can be restored when needed. Sometimes it is practical to use removable hard disks, permitting several copies of the operating system to be available should they be needed.

SUMMARY

Computer systems are an essential part of a functioning nuclear medicine facility. The rapid development of hardware and sophisticated software has led to imaging studies of great clinical usefulness. As a result, it is necessary for the nuclear medicine specialist to maintain familiarity with the systems that provide the clinical images for interpretation.

ANNOTATED BIBLIOGRAPHY

General and Nonimaging Instruments

1. Sorenson JA, Phelps ME. *Physics in Nuclear Medicine.* 2nd ed. Orlando: Grune and Stratton, 1987.

   This classic physics and instrumentation textbook provides an excellent introduction to the theory of nonimaging and imaging instrumentation.

2. Attix FH. *Introduction to Radiological Physics and Radiation Dosimetry.* New York: Wiley, 1986.

The definite textbook of the underlying physics of radiation detectors and dose-measuring instruments (not for the mathematically shy or faint-hearted).

3. Knoll GF. *Radiation Detection and Measurement.* 2nd ed. New York: Wiley, 1989.
   Comprehensive textbook on detector technology and electronics. Written for upper division college or first-year graduate students in nuclear engineering or medical physics.

Anger Cameras

4. Graham LS. Clinically applicable modifications of Anger camera technology. In: Freeman LM, Weissmann HS, eds. *Nuclear Medicine Annual 1983.* New York: Raven Press, 1983:51–96.
   A summary of the technical improvements in scintillation cameras as of 1983.

5. Hoffer PB, Neumann R, Quartararo L, et al. Improved intrinsic resolution: does it make a difference? *J Nucl Med* 1984;25:230–236.
   A study of the effect of improving intrinsic spatial resolution. No significant difference in the spatial resolution of clinical studies was observed.

6. La Fontaine R, Stein MA, Graham LS, et al. Cold lesions: enhanced contrast using asymmetric photopeak windows. *Radiology* 1986;160:255–260.
   Analyzer windows that are set on the high side of the photopeak provide improved contrast and lesion detectability with an increase in imaging time.

7. Muehllehner G, Colsher JG, Stoub EW. Correction of field nonuniformity in scintigraphic cameras through removal of spatial distortion. *J Nucl Med* 1980;21:771–776.

8. Stoub EW, Colsher JG, Lee PC, et al. A spatial distortion correction method for gamma cameras. *J Nucl Med* 1979;20:608.
   Description of the techniques that are used to correct for spatial distortion in scintillation cameras.

9. Patton JJ, Rollo FD, Brill AB. Recent developments in nuclear medicine instrumentation. *IEEE Trans Nucl Sci* 1980;NS-27:1066–1072.
   A technical review of developments in imaging instrumentation as of 1980.

10. Royal HD, Parker JA, Kolodny GM. Noncardiac, nontomographic applications of the slant-hole collimator. *J Nucl Med* 1982;23:786–789.
   A description of clinical applications of the slant-hole collimator.

11. White W. Resolution, sensitivity, and contrast in gamma-camera design: a critical review. *Radiology* 1979;132:179–187.
   A review of the state-of-the-art in scintillation cameras as of 1979.

12. Beck RN, Zimmer LT, Charleston DB, et al. A theory of optimum utilization of all detected radiation. In: *Semiconductor Detectors in Medicine.* CONF-730321. Oak Ridge, TN, U.S. Atomic Energy Commission Technical Information Center, 1973:88–106.
   A description of the theory behind the use of energy-weighted acquisition imaging.

Quality Control

13. AAPM Report No. 6: *Scintillation Camera Acceptance Testing and Performance Evaluation.* New York: American Institute of Physics, 1980.
   A comprehensive description of noncomputerized tests that can be used for evaluation of Anger camera performance.

14. Chapman DR, Garcia EV, Waxman AD. Misalignment of multiple photopeak analyzer outputs: effects on imaging. *J Nucl Med* 1980;21:872–874.
   Superimposed flood field images taken at different energies with gallium-67 can be used as a quality control procedure to assess multiple-window spatial registration errors.

15. Graham LS. Quality assurance of Anger cameras. In: Rao DV, Chandra R, Graham MC, eds. *Physics of Nuclear Medicine: Recent Advances.* New York: American Institute of Physics, 1983:68–83.

A description of basic quality control procedures for all important performance parameters for Anger scintillation cameras.

16. *Workshop Manual for Quality Control of Scintillation Cameras in Nuclear Medicine.* HEW Publication (FDA) No. 76-8039. U.S. Department of Health, Education, and Welfare, 1976.

Procedures are given for performing and evaluating routine quality control procedures on Anger scintillation cameras.

Single-Photon Emission Computed Tomography and Positron Emission Tomography

17. Jaszczak RJ, Murphy PH, Huard D, Burdine JA. Radionuclide emission computed tomography of the head with Tc-99m and a scintillation camera. *J Nucl Med* 1977;18:373–380.

An early report demonstrating SPECT imaging with a rotation Anger camera using a filtered backprojection reconstruction algorithm.

18. Rogers WL, Clinthorne NH, Harkness BA, Koral KF, Keyes JW Jr. Field-flood requirements for emission computed tomography with an Anger camera. *J Nucl Med* 1982;23:162–168.

This report demonstrates that uniformity correction using field floods requires many millions of counts to improve uniformity; otherwise, circular artifacts are introduced.

19. Gottschalk SC, Salem D, Lim CB, Wake RH. SPECT resolution and uniformity improvements by noncircular orbit. *J Nucl Med* 1983;24:822–828.

Noncircular orbits are useful in body SPECT imaging; improved resolution is due to closer spacing between body and collimator than can be obtained with circular orbits.

20. Tamaki N, Mukai T, Ishii Y, et al. Comparative study of thallium emission myocardial tomography with 180° and 360° data collection. *J Nucl Med* 1982;23:661–666.

Many reports have been published that compare 180° and 360° data collection in thallium SPECT imaging of the heart. The conclusions of these reports are not in agreement. However, in practice it appears that 180° data collection is gaining acceptance.

21. Jaszczak RJ, Chang L-T, Murphy PH. Single photon emission computed tomography using multi-slice fan-beam collimators. *IEEE Trans Nucl Sci* 1979;NS-26:610–618.

This early report described the successful implementation of a fan-beam collimator for SPECT imaging. It was nearly a decade before these collimators and the associated reconstruction algorithms became commercially successful.

22. King MA, Schwinger RB, Penney BC. Variation of the count-dependent Metz filter with imaging system modulation transfer function. *Med Phys* 1986;13:139–149.

Visual interpretation of computed images is influenced by the structure of the noise. The appearance of noise can be altered by filtering to minimize its influence on interpretation.

23. Borello JA, Clinthorne NH, Rogers WL, Thrall JH, Keyes JW Jr. Oblique-angle tomography: a restructuring algorithm for transaxial tomographic data. *J Nucl Med* 1981;22:471–473.

Particularly in cardiac imaging, it is important to be able to reslice the data after acquisition and reconstruction to align the image planes with anatomic directions, such as the major axis of the heart. This can be performed with little or no loss of image quality because rotating Anger camera SPECT systems have nearly equal resolution and fine sampling in all directions.

24. Chang L-T. A method for attenuation correction in radionuclide computed tomography. *IEEE Trans Nucl Sci* 1978;NS-25:638–643.

The "Chang" method of attenuation correction described in this report is widely implemented in commercially available scanners.

25. Jaszczak RJ, Greer KL, Floyd CE Jr, Harris CC, Coleman RE. Improved SPECT quantification using compensation for scattered photons. *J Nucl Med* 1984;25:893–900.

Scattered photons produce a background in reconstructed images that makes accurate quantitation difficult. The described method of scatter correction significantly improves quantitation in SPECT imaging.

26. Lim CB, Walker R, Pinkstaff C, et al. Triangular SPECT system for 3-D total organ volume imaging: performance results and dynamic imaging capability. *IEEE Trans Nucl Sci* 1986;NS-33:501–504.

By means of three detectors, the brain can be completely surrounded with detectors, yet the detectors can be moved apart radially to permit body imaging.

27. Rogers WL, Clinthorne NH, Stamos J, et al. Performance evaluation of SPRINT, a single photon ring tomograph for brain imaging. *J Nucl Med* 1984;25:1013–1018.

The approach described in this report demonstrates a system configuration that is optimized for SPECT imaging. The detectors are stationary, and only the collimator rotates.

28. Kirsch C-M, Moore SC, Zimmerman RE, English RJ, Holman BL. Characteristics of a scanning, multidetector, single photon ECT body imager. *J Nucl Med* 1981;22:726–731.

The multidetector dedicated SPECT scanner described in this report uses a scanning motion and highly focused collimators. Its unique characteristic is that it images a single slice but with very high sensitivity.

29. Stokely EM, Sveinsdottir E, Lassen NA, Rommer P. A single photon dynamic computer assisted tomograph (DCAT) for imaging brain function in multiple cross-sections. *J Comput Assist Tomogr* 1980;4:230–240.

This report describes a dedicated multicrystal SPECT scanner specifically designed for fast dynamic imaging.

30. Bohm C, Eriksson L, Bergstrom M, Litton J, Sundman R, Singh M. A computer assisted ring detector positron camera system for reconstruction tomography of the brain. *IEEE Trans Nucl Sci* 1978;NS-25;624–637.

An early report describing a PET scanner similar to others designed and built during the same period.

31. Hoffman EJ, Phelps ME, Huang SC, et al. ECAT III—a new PET system for heart and whole body dynamic imaging. *J Nucl Med* 1985;26:p28.

The PET scanner described in this report has very good spatial resolution and gives images of remarkable quality. More recent designs have mainly focused on using position encoding to simplify the design.

32. Karp JS, Muehllehner G, Mankoff DA, et al. Continuous-slice PENN-PET: a positron tomograph with volume-imaging capability. *J Nucl Med* (in press).

The PET scanner described in this report is designed for clinical use and has very closely spaced (2 mm) slices, allowing calculation of sagittal, coronal, and oblique views without sampling problems.

Computer Terminology and Hardware

33. Cradduck TD, Busemann-Sokole E. Computers in nuclear medicine. *Radiographics* 1985;5:52–82.

Good overview of computers applied to nuclear medicine. Good list of desirable features when selecting computers. Provides recommendations for quality assurance programs.

34. Erickson JJ. Nuclear medicine computer hardware. In: Erickson JJ, Rollo FD, eds. *Digital Nuclear Medicine.* Philadelphia: J.B. Lippincott, 1983: 47–59.
Good, broad review of computer hardware. Some of the material is out of date.

35. Simmons GH, Kereiakes JG, Pickens DR, Erickson JJ. Computer hardware and software fundamentals. *Radiographics* 1985;5:11–30.
Introductory description of general computer hardware and software.

36. Pickens DR, Erickson JJ. Computers in computed tomography and magnetic resonance imaging. *Radiographics* 1985;5:31–50.
Introductory description of computer hardware for computed tomographic and magnetic resonance imaging. Includes description of array processors, image display systems, ADCs, and digital-to-analog converters.

37. Erickson JJ, Pickens DR. Signal processing. In: Williams LE, ed. *Nuclear Medical Physics.* Boca Raton, FL: CRC Press, 1987:39–57.
Descriptions of array processors, ADCs, computer bus, and digital displays for use in nuclear medicine.

38. Erickson JJ. Quality control of nuclear medicine computer systems. In: Erickson JJ, Rollo FD, eds. *Digital Nuclear Medicine.* Philadelphia: J.B. Lippincott, 1983:47–59.
Good introduction to quality assurance issues.

Computer Systems for Single-Photon Emission Computed Tomography

39. Keyes JW Jr. Instrumentation. In: Ell PJ, Holman BL, eds. *Computed Emission Tomography.* New York: Oxford University Press 1982:243–262.
Describes SPECT instrumentation. Good, brief description of the computer used in performing SPECT studies.

40. Croft BY. *Single-Photon Emission Computed Tomography.* Chicago: Year Book Medical Publishers, Inc., 1986.
Description of all aspects of SPECT. Good description of instrumentation, computer requirements, and quality assurance. General descriptions of clinical applications.

41. Todd-Pokropek AE, Jarritt PH. The noise characteristics of SPECT systems. In: Ell PJ, Holman BL, eds. *Computed Emission Tomography.* New York: Oxford University Press, 1982:361–389.
Mathematical descriptions of noise sources in SPECT imaging. Includes descriptions of reconstruction filter characteristics.

Computer Software

42. Pickens DR. The operating system. In: Erickson JJ, Rollo FD, eds. *Digital Nuclear Medicine.* Philadelphia: J.B. Lippincott, 1983:60–80.
Very broad review of operating systems and their designs. Additional brief discussion of languages and programming.

43. Hunter TB, ed. *The Computer in Radiology.* Rockville, MD: Aspen Systems Corp, 1986.
Detailed description of computer hardware and software; chapters 1–5 by different authors.

Nuclear Medicine Software

44. Gelfand MJ, Thomas SR, eds. *Effective Use of Computers in Nuclear Medicine.* New York: McGraw-Hill, 1988.
Excellent, detailed descriptions of acquisition and processing using computers in a nuclear medicine laboratory. Includes extensive chapters on SPECT acquisition and processing. Probably the best collected reference work of computer use in nuclear medicine imaging.

45. Villanueva-Meyer J, Philippe L, Cordero S, Marcus CS, Mena I. Use of factor analysis in the evaluation of left to right shunts. *J Nucl Med* 1986;27:1442–1448.

Comparison of factor analysis with standard manual ROI methods for cardiac shunt evaluation.

46. Eisner R, Churchwell A, Noever T, et al. Quantitative analysis of the tomographic thallium-201 myocardial bullseye display: critical role of correcting for patient motion. *J Nucl Med* 1988;29:91–97.

Description of bullseye presentation of SPECT thallium-201 images and the effects of small amounts of patient motion on the display. Discussion of motion correction algorithm applied to image set before display.

47. Cavailloles F, Bazin J-P, Di Paola R. Factor analysis in gated cardiac studies. *J Nucl Med* 1984;25:1067–1079.

Extensive mathematical description of factor analysis of dynamic structures. Comparison of the method with Fourier analysis in 45 gated cardiac studies. Four-color illustrations.

48. Garcia EV, Train KV, Maddahi J, et al. Quantification of rotational thallium-201 myocardial tomography. *J Nucl Med* 1985;26:17–26.

Detailed description of the Cedars-Sinai SPECT thallium-201 quantitation programs with clinical results.

49. Jones JP. Nuclear medicine operating systems. In: Erickson JJ, Rollo FD, eds. *Digital Nuclear Medicine.* Philadelphia: J.B. Lippincott, 1983:81–93.

Brief description of acquisition software systems as well as a description of typical collection techniques.

50. Jones JP. Clinical imaging studies. In: Erickson JJ, Rollo FD, eds. *Digital Nuclear Medicine.* Philadelphia: J.B. Lippincott, 1983:105–154.

Description of most of the usual methods of data analysis of nuclear medicine images. Includes heart studies of various types, lung perfusion studies, and renal studies.

51. Byron E, Pavel DG, Swiryn S, Mayer-Pavel C. Phase images of gated cardiac studies: a standard evaluation procedure. In: Esser PD, ed. *Functional Mapping of Organ Systems.* New York: Society of Nuclear Medicine, 1982:129–138.

Description of Fourier analysis of cardiac images, including mathematics.

52. Rabinowitz A, Wexler JP, Blaufox MD. Quantification of the radionuclide image: theoretical concepts and the role of the computer. In: Freeman LM, ed. *Freeman and Johnson's Clinical Radionuclide Imaging.* New York: Grune and Stratton, 1984:261–313.

Good description of computer hardware, acquisition software, and general analysis software. Concise presentation.

53. Patton DD. Computers in nuclear medicine. In: Hunter TB, ed. *The Computer in Radiology.* Rockville, MD: Aspen, 1986:178–205.

Broad discussion of acquisition and processing software for nuclear medicine.

Multiple-Choice Questions

DIRECTIONS

Items 1–11 consist of a question or an incomplete statement followed by four or five lettered answers or completions. Select the one lettered answer or completion that is best in each case, and fill in the circle containing the corresponding letter on the answer sheet.

1. Which one of the following is *NOT* a characteristic of an ionization chamber survey meter?

A. Significantly less energy dependence than a Geiger-Mueller survey meter
B. Ability to measure high exposure rates
C. Costs roughly the same as a Geiger-Mueller survey meter
D. Instrument of choice for measuring exposure rates for a patient treated with iodine-131 for thyroid carcinoma
E. Production of very small currents when exposed to radiation

2. A dose calibrator linearity check was performed by repetitive counting of a technetium generator elution that was reserved for this purpose (Table 1). Which statement *best* describes the result?

A. Linearity is acceptable throughout the entire activity range tested.
B. Linearity is acceptable from the lowest activities tested up to and including an indicated reading of 20,000 MBq.
C. Linearity above 10,000 MBq is unacceptable, but no correction factors are needed at these high activities because aliquots drawn from these high-activity vials are always in the activity range where linearity is acceptable.
D. Linearity up to and including 10,000 MBq is acceptable, but correction factors must be determined for higher activities.
E. Linearity is unacceptable above about 10,000 MBq and below about 37 MBq.

Table 1

Elapsed Time (hr)	Activity Reading (MBq)
0	30,000
6	17,800
12	9,700
18	5,000
24	2,550
36	620
48	154

3. The major purpose of automatic tuning circuits in scintillation cameras is to

A. decrease maintenance costs.
B. increase the lifetime of photomultiplier tubes (PMTs).
C. improve intrinsic spatial resolution.
D. maintain the integrity of energy and linearity correction maps.
E. eliminate the need for routine quality control tests.

4. The removal of scattered photons during the process of image formation will

A. improve the contrast in clinical images.
B. reduce imaging time.

C. decrease the statistical fluctuations (noise) in an image.
D. improve camera energy resolution.
E. improve camera field uniformity.

5. Which *one* of the following is *NOT* used to improve count rate performance of scintillation cameras?

A. Derandomizer buffers
B. Dual-integrator circuits
C. Pileup rejection circuits
D. Energy-weighted acquisition
E. Decreased integration time

6. When energy registration (multiple-window spatial registration) errors are present in a camera, which *one* of the following occurs?

A. Resolving (dead) time increases.
B. Spatial resolution improves.
C. Contrast is lost.
D. Spatial distortion occurs.
E. Energy resolution deteriorates.

7. Which *one* of the following represents the primary purpose of a noncircular or elliptic scanning motion in single-photon emission computed tomographic (SPECT) imaging?

A. Improved spatial resolution
B. Easier patient positioning
C. Improved sensitivity
D. Easier implementation of attenuation correction algorithm
E. Easier implementation of the backprojection algorithm

8. Which *one* of the following statements concerning a cone-beam SPECT study is true?

A. The collimator scans linearly.
B. The detector is stationary, but the collimator moves.
C. The collimator rotates around its own axis.
D. It provides a several-fold increase in sensitivity compared with a parallel-hole collimator.
E. Reconstruction times for cone-beam SPECT are comparable to those for routine SPECT imaging.

9. Your computer system requires a major service call for failure of the camera interface. At the same time, the service representative installs the latest upgrade of the operating system and the application programs. After the representative leaves, you should instruct your technologist to perform which *one* of the following operations?

A. Begin patient studies.
B. Perform routine quality assurance tests.
C. Back up the software and perform routine quality assurance tests.

D. Perform a series of validation studies.
E. Analyze unprocessed data.

10. A sudden reduced intensity defect in the center of a bladder image during an effective renal plasma flow study is most likely caused by which *one* of the following?

A. Hard disk error
B. Memory error
C. Software error
D. Overflow error
E. Analysis error

11. The image shown in Figure 1 is an example of which *one* of the following?

A. Patient movement during data acquisition
B. Faulty analog-to-digital converter
C. Using a low-energy collimator to image a patient containing a radionuclide that emits high-energy photons
D. Multiple-window spatial registration error
E. Faulty electronic formatter

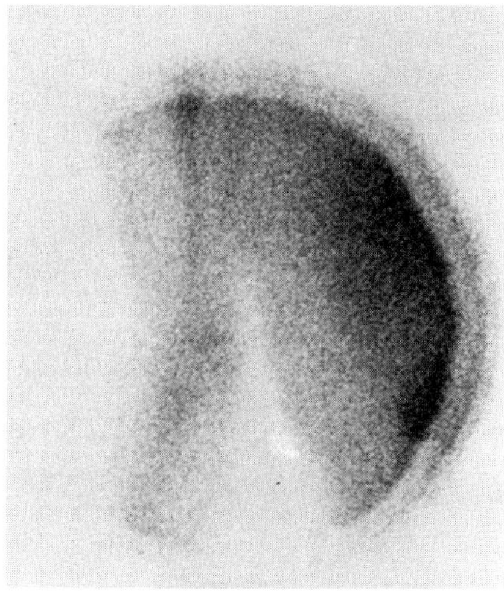

Figure 1

DIRECTIONS

Items 12–47 consist of five lettered headings followed by a list of numbered phrases or statements. For *each* numbered phrase or statement, select the *one* lettered heading that is *most* closely associated with it and fill in the circle containing the corresponding letter on the answer sheet. *Each lettered heading may be selected once, more than once, or not at all.*

For each instrument described (items 12–16), select the appropriate instrument type (options A–E).

A. Geiger-Mueller survey meter
B. Ionization chamber survey meter
C. Radionuclide (dose) calibrator
D. Sodium iodide [NaI(Tl)] counting system
E. High-purity germanium semiconductor detector

12. Preferred instrument for counting indium-111 mixed with technetium-99m in a blood sample
13. Preferred instrument for measuring exposure rate inside a radioactive waste storage area filled with jugs of urine collected from patients treated for thyroid carcinoma with iodine-131
14. Instrument capable of displaying activity readings in units of gigabecquerels
15. Instrument that uses a reentrant-well detector configuration exclusively
16. Instrument that exhibits large dead time and thus can be used only for low count rate applications

For each of the following quality control tests for scintillation cameras (items 17–21), select the recommended frequency of performance (options A–E).

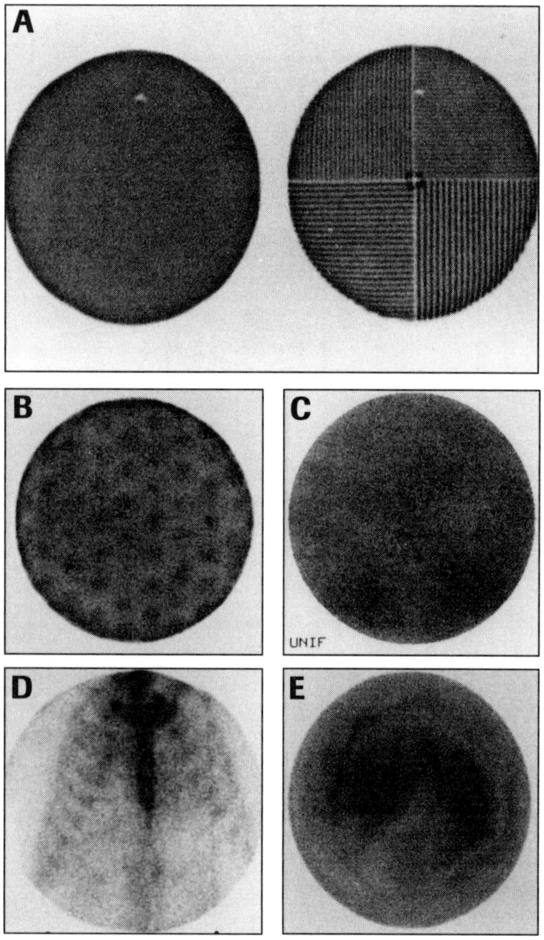

Figures 2A-E

A. Daily
B. Weekly
C. Monthly
D. Quarterly
E. Annually

17. Field uniformity
18. Linearity
19. Maximum count rate
20. Multiple-window spatial registration
21. Sensitivity

For each of the examples of nonuniformity shown in Figure 2 (items 22–26), select the most appropriate explanation (options A–E).

A. Photomultiplier tube(s) out of tune
B. Pulse height analyzer window set off-peak
C. Cracked crystal
D. Analog-to-digital converter artifact
E. Nonuniform liquid-filled flood

22. Figure 2A
23. Figure 2B
24. Figure 2C
25. Figure 2D
26. Figure 2E

Select the most appropriate choice (options A–D) for each imaging parameter (items 27–29).

A. Single-photon emission computed tomographic imaging
B. Positron emission tomographic imaging
C. Both
D. Neither

27. Improved image contrast compared with planar (two-dimensional) imaging
28. Accurate quantitation of in vivo distribution of radioactive tracer
29. Attenuation correction usually performed, most often with a transmission scan

Select the most appropriate instrument (options A–E) for each descriptive statement (items 30–33).

A. Dedicated SPECT scanner with annular crystal
B. Rotating Anger camera with single detector
C. Rotating Anger camera with two or three detectors
D. B and C
E. A, B, and C

30. The detector is stationary, and only the collimator rotates.
31. The device can be used equally well for brain and body imaging.

32. The device can be used with fan-beam collimators.
33. The detectors should be as close as possible to the patient for best spatial resolution.

For each characteristic (items 34–37), select the most appropriate computer component (options A–E).

A. Optical disk
B. Random access memory
C. Hard disk
D. Cache memory
E. Floppy disk

34. Directly related to the available temporal resolution of gated cardiac studies
35. Directly related to the number of studies that can be stored during a day's clinical activity
36. Directly related to archival storage of large numbers of images
37. Directly related to increased speed of collection and analysis

For each acquisition mode (items 38–42), select the most appropriate use (options A–E).

A. Static acquisition
B. Gated list mode acquisition
C. Dynamic acquisition
D. Gated acquisition
E. List mode acquisition

38. First-pass cardiac studies
39. Rest ventriculogram using technetium-99m–labeled red blood cells
40. Renal function studies
41. Liver imaging
42. Cardiac studies in the presence of arrhythmias

For each functional description (items 43–47), select the most appropriate technique (options A–E).

A. Deconvolution
B. Filtering
C. Edge detection
D. Phase analysis
E. Backprojection

43. Reduces a gated cardiac study to a more compact form (functional image) before interpretation
44. Makes use of the first harmonic component to represent motion and timing of a cardiac study
45. Is used to select a region of an image for processing
46. Can be used in dynamic studies to compute an approximation of an instantaneous arrival of a tracer bolus in the organ of interest
47. Can be used to remove noise from an image

DIRECTIONS

Items 48–150 consist of a heading followed by a number of statements related to that heading. Mark each of the numbered statements as true or false.

Important properties of well ionization chambers (radionuclide calibrators) that utilize pressurized argon (unlike nonpressurized systems) include which of the following?

48. Higher sensitivity at low activity levels
49. Less dependence on geometry
50. Ability to measure larger volume samples
51. Larger currents produced for the same activity level
52. Accuracy less affected by the presence of a high room background

Features of NaI(Tl) well detectors especially designed to provide optimum operation and maximum counting efficiency include which of the following?

53. Protective casing of lead surrounding the crystal to prevent the entrance of stray light
54. Crystal shape giving almost 4-*p* counting geometry
55. Coupling of the crystal and PMT to prevent light loss
56. Hermetically sealed crystal
57. Absence of preamplifiers from most counting systems

True statements regarding the use of constancy tests in the quality control of a radionuclide calibrator include which of the following?

58. They must be performed each day that the radionuclide calibrator is used.
59. They must be performed for all commonly used radionuclide settings.
60. The radionuclide used for the constancy test must be one of those used for clinical studies.
61. The radionuclide calibrator must be repaired or replaced if the error is greater than 610%.

True statements concerning liquid scintillation counters include which of the following?

62. The material to be counted is dissolved or dispersed in the counting fluid.
63. Depending on the material to be counted, different types of counting fluid may be used.
64. All counting fluids are water soluble.
65. Because of variations in counting efficiency, most counting systems calculate correction factors to facilitate data analysis.
66. Modern liquid scintillation counters are operated at refrigerator temperatures to minimize thermionic noise.

A 1000-channel multichannel analyzer (MCA) is used with a 7.5-cm NaI(Tl) well detector to count serum samples in small test tubes for technetium-99m–labeled (DTPA) glomerular filtration rate [GFR] and iodine-131–labeled orthoiodohippurate (effective renal plasma flow [ERPF]). The MCA is calibrated for 1,000-keV full scale, and symmetric windows for technetium-99m, iodine-131, and cesium-137 are set. True statements concerning multi-channel analyzers include which of the following?

67. Energy calibration should be verified by adjusting the amplifier gain so that the photopeak from a cesium-137 rod source inserted in the well is centered in channel 662.
68. The activity of the cesium-137 rod source must be recalculated daily for use in performing the day-to-day constancy check.
69. The activity of the cesium-137 rod source does not need to be recalculated daily for use in calibrating the amplifier gain, or kiloelectron volts per channel.
70. The resolution of a 1,000-channel MCA is so good that correction for downscatter of iodine-131 photons into the technetium-99m window is not necessary when counting samples containing both radionuclides.
71. A good check to ensure that the well has not become contaminated from patient samples would be to obtain a 10-min background count in the cesium-137 window.

A NaI(Tl) well counter is used to count samples collected during a GFR study performed with 500 MBq (1.35 mCi) of technetium-99m–labeled DTPA. Blood samples are collected in 7-ml evacuated tubes that are allowed to fill until the vacuum is exhausted. Urine samples are pipetted into similar tubes. True statements include which of the following?

72. There may be detrimental dead-time losses if the blood samples are counted immediately at the end of the 2-hr collection period.
73. After correction for radioactive decay and dead time, a fully mixed whole-blood tube (7 ml) counted immediately at the end of the study and then counted again the next day without resuspension of the red cells in the serum will yield the same count rate.
74. If dead-time losses are too great to allow reliable corrections, the tubes may be counted several centimeters above the face of the detector to take advantage of the drastic drop in count rate when a sample is not in the well.
75. If the usual volume of serum is 4 ml, but one of the blood samples yielded only 1 ml of serum, it is accurate to simply multiply the count rate by a factor of 4 to make it equivalent to the 4-ml samples.
76. Dead-time losses can be eliminated or reduced by narrowing the window until the recorded count rate has dropped into the "safe" range for the instrument.

Uniformity correction techniques that minimize the fundamental causes of nonuniformity include which of the following?

77. Count skimming
78. Count addition
79. Distortion correction
80. Energy correction
81. Unblank modulation

In recent years, the intrinsic spatial resolution of scintillation cameras has been improved by which of the following changes?

82. Decreasing the unblank time
83. Decreasing the thickness of light pipes
84. Increasing the number of PMTs
85. Using thin-walled foil collimators
86. Using distortion correction circuits

Moving the pulse height analyzer windows slightly to the high side of the photopeak in a scintillation camera achieves which of the following?

87. Increased count rate
88. Improved field uniformity
89. Decreased number of scattered photons that are used in forming the image
90. Increased sensitivity for dynamic studies
91. Improved energy registration

Substitution of a converging collimator for a parallel-hole collimator results in which of the following?

92. Spatial resolution falls off less rapidly with distance from the face of the collimator
93. Field-of-view increases
94. Clinical images are often distorted
95. Counting efficiency is increased for small target organs

Image contrast in scintillation camera images can be improved by

96. Off-peak imaging.
97. Using a detector with better energy resolution.
98. Energy-weighted acquisition.
99. Increasing the window size.
100. Using a low-resolution collimator.

Smart consoles for scintillation cameras can be used to do which of the following?

101. Set up predefined protocols.
102. Adjust the display for different types of film.
103. Apply energy correction to clinical images.
104. Apply distortion correction to clinical images.
105. Perform simple analyses of clinical studies.

True statements regarding positron emission tomographic (PET) imaging include which of the following?

106. By eliminating the collimator, PET scanners can achieve better spatial resolution than SPECT scanners.
107. The point of origin of the annihilation quanta is determined by using mechanical collimation.
108. Better spatial resolution can only be achieved by sacrificing sensitivity.
109. Positron emission tomographic scanners have both better spatial resolution and better sensitivity than SPECT systems

True statements concerning SPECT imaging include which of the following?

110. Spatial resolution is best near the center of the field-of-view in the transverse plane.
111. Single-photon emission tomographic imaging provides higher image contrast than planar imaging.
112. Single-photon emission tomographic imaging requires certain quality control procedures not needed for planar imaging.

113. Separate data acquisitions are necessary for transverse, sagittal and coronal views.

True statements concerning SPECT attenuation correction include which of the following?

114. The body contour can be defined with a transmission study.
115. Determining the attenuation coefficients with a transmission scan is more accurate than assuming a constant attenuation coefficient.
116. Cardiac SPECT scanning with 180° data collection makes attenuation correction more difficult.
117. Attenuation correction reduces spatial resolution.

Which of the following generally degrades image quality in SPECT studies?

118. Changes in PMT output in response to changing PMT orientation in the earth's magnetic field
119. Center-of-rotation errors
120. Use of high-count flood correction
121. Nonlinearity (distortion) in the scintillation detector

The artifact that appears in the transverse section of the liver shown in Figure 3 could be produced by which of the following?

122. Incorrect center-of-rotation calibration
123. Movement of the patient during acquisition of the images
124. A nonuniformity in the detector
125. A nonuniformity in the collimator
126. Reconstruction with a Parzen filter

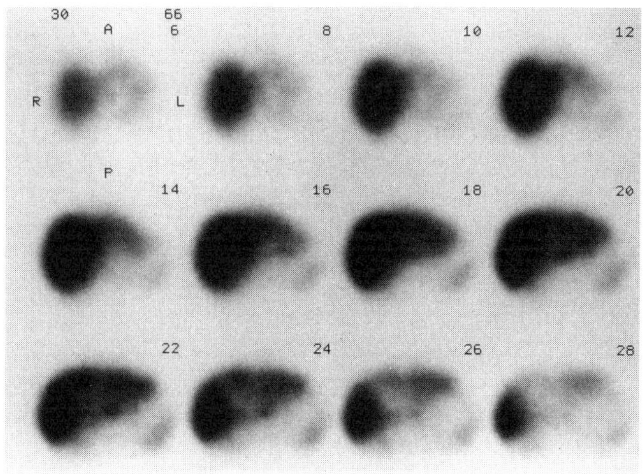

Figure 3

Which of the following functions are provided by the operating system of a nuclear medicine computer?

127. Calculation of ejection fraction curves
128. Communication with the user
129. Recordkeeping of disk and memory usage
130. Information processing from ADCs
131. Displaying SPECT cardiac images

A time–activity curve displaying tracer concentration in a target organ (other than the heart or aorta) is produced from a dynamic acquisition. True statements concerning postprocessing operations that can be used to decrease random noise in the data include which of the following?

132. The curve can be processed with a running-average filter.
133. The curve can be fitted with an exponential function.
134. The curve can be deconvolved with a time–activity curve from the aorta.
135. The curve can be processed with a low-pass Fourier transform filter.
136. The curve can be processed with a high-pass filter.

True statements concerning operations that can be performed by ADCs in a nuclear medicine computer include which of the following?

137. They can reduce the field-of-view of an image.
138. They can compare two numbers and make a choice.
139. They can reconstruct images.
140. They can cause artifacts due to drift and other instabilities.
141. They store images for later processing.

You are asked to help select a computer system that will be used with a rotating-camera SPECT system. The camera and computer will be used to generate both conventional static images of various organs and tomographic images of the brain and liver. The minimum requirements for an effective system include which of the following?

142. Electrocardiographic inputs
143. Hard disk drive
144. Array processor
145. Large memory
146. Optical disk

True statements concerning analyzing image data include which of the following?

147. Thresholding permanently changes the appearance of images.
148. Filtering an image with a five-point smoothing filter improves the spatial resolution of the image.
149. Filtering images with a Fourier transform filter requires more time than filtering operations with non-Fourier filters.
150. Temporal filtering is done to reduce noise in dynamic data sets.

Answers, Critiques, and References for Multiple-Choice Questions

ITEM 1: CHARACTERISTICS OF SURVEY METERS

Answer: *C*

The detector of an ionization chamber survey meter operates in the ionization chamber region of the gas-filled detector characteristic curve. In this region, the number of ion pairs collected is equal to the number of ion pairs generated in the gas, (i.e., the multiplication factor is 1). Because of the low density of the gas in the counting chamber, very few ion pairs are created when a single gamma ray traverses the chamber. Detection of the tiny electrical currents created by such a small number of ion pairs is very difficult. Hence, ionization chamber survey meters do not attempt to count the individual gamma rays; rather, they are designed to measure the essentially continuous electrical current created when large numbers of gamma rays per second interact with the gas in the chamber. Indeed, the ionization chamber survey meter is ideally suited for measuring very large exposure rates because it has essentially no dead time and gives a linear response up to high exposure rates, such as would be encountered in the vicinity of a patient with a thyroid carcinoma or other high-activity source.

Geiger-Mueller (G-M) survey meters operate in the region of the gas-filled detector characteristic curve where the multiplication factor is on the order of 1 million or more. In this region, a single ion pair causes millions of electrons to be collected, producing a large pulse that is easily detected by rather simple, rugged, inexpensive electronics. The electronics associated with an ionization chamber survey meter must operate at low electrical currents and are substantially more expensive than G-M survey meter electronics. Thus, the cost of an ionization chamber survey meter may be two or three times higher than the cost a G-M survey meter.

Another consequence of the operation of a detector in the G-M region of the gas-filled detector characteristic curve is that the detector gives off a large pulse regardless of whether the incident gamma ray imparts low or high kinetic energy to the liberated ion pair. If a low-energy gamma ray possesses sufficient energy to penetrate the metal wall or entrance window of a G-M detector, it can cause a pulse to be generated and detected. In the ionization chamber, however, the low-energy gamma ray may impart so little kinetic energy to the liberated ion pair that recombination can occur before the ion pair can be collected. Thus, the ionization chamber survey meter exhibits falsely low readings for low-energy gamma rays to an extent that is far greater than that for a G-M survey meter. However, over a wide range of photon energies, ionization chambers measure exposure rates in (mR/hr or coulombs/kg) in a way that is markedly less dependent on the energy of the photons than G-M survey meters.

ITEM 2: RADIONUCLIDE CALIBRATOR LINEARITY CHECK

Answer: *D*

If the activity readings are graphed, there is a significant departure from linearity above about 10,000 MBq and good linearity throughout the remainder of the range below 10,000 MBq. Review of Table I reveals that the 12-hr reading of roughly 10,000 MBq is within the ±5% tolerance for the linearity, but the 0- and 6-hr readings are not within the tolerance. A clinic might choose never to measure the total activity of an elution vial to keep all their measurements within the linear region. This would require withdrawing an accurately measured volume of eluate for assay, an operation that would subject the technologist or radiopharmacist to an unnecessary radiation dose. Further, there would need to be an administrative prohibition against using the calibrator for activities exceeding 10,000 MBq; such an administrative requirement would be difficult to monitor, and its violation could lead to excessive handling of stock vials and excessive radiation doses to workers.

ITEM 3: AUTOMATIC TUNING OF SCINTILLATION CAMERAS

Answer: *D*

A change in the balance of the photomultiplier tubes (PMTs) in a camera modifies the energy and linearity correction factors that are used to produce a uniform flood field image. For example, if the voltage of a PMT in a camera that does not have automatic tuning increases, more counts are pulled into the area associated with that tube, and a hot spot is created. This condition can only be corrected by readjusting the voltage of the tube or by preparing a new correction map. The simplest approach is to monitor the response of each tube and adjust its gain or high voltage as needed to maintain field uniformity. Microprocessors perform this function in many state-of-the-art cameras. A comprehensive quality control program is needed to guarantee the user that

Table I

Elapsed Time (hr)	Activity reading (MBq)	Time Multiplier	Expected reading (MBq)	Deviation
0	30,000	256×	39,424	−23.1
6	17,800	128×	19,712	−9.7
12	9,700	64×	9,856	−1.6
18	5,000	32×	4,928	+1.5
24	2,550	16×	2,464	+3.5
36	620	4×	616	+0.6
48	154	1×	154	0.0

the energy and linearity corrections are working properly. If anything, these circuits add one more layer of complexity to an instrument that is already quite sophisticated.

Although automatic tuning may reduce the number of service calls required to "tune" the PMTs, that is not its primary purpose. Random fluctuation of PMT voltage is normal, and there is some change in performance with age. However, these have no effect on overall lifetime of the PMTs.

A poorly balanced camera may show a slight loss of spatial resolution, but the possibility of producing artifacts due to the presence of areas of increased or decreased activity is a more serious problem.

REFERENCES

1. Graham LS. Clinically applicable modifications of Anger camera technology. In: Freeman LM, Weissmann HS, eds. *Nuclear Medicine Annual 1983.* New York: Raven Press, 1983:51–96.
2. Graham LS. Automatic tuning of scintillation cameras: a review. *J Nucl Med Tech* 1986; 14:105–110.

ITEM 4: EFFECT OF REMOVING SCATTERED PHOTONS

Answer: *A*

Image quality is degraded by the presence of scattered photons, and 15% to 20% windows have been found to be a reasonable compromise between the desire to obtain as many counts as possible and the degradation associated with the inclusion of scattered photons. If a 20% window is used for technetium-99m, photons may be scattered by as much as 55° and still be accepted. Scattered photons decrease contrast by producing a general background that is superimposed on the image produced by photons that have not been scattered. Removal of these photons by the use of narrower analyzer windows, off-peak imaging, or deconvolution increases contrast.

Because the first two techniques reduce the number of photons passed by the pulse-height analyzer, a longer time is required to collect the same total number of usable photons. If acquisition time is not increased, the statistical fluctuations will be larger (more noise). Even when the total number of counts in the image is held constant, the noise level will never be better than when scatter elimination techniques are not used.

Energy resolution is a measure of the ability of a detector system to accurately determine the energy of the incident photons. The smaller the energy resolution (expressed as a percent of the photopeak energy), the more accurate it is. By definition, removing scattered radiation does not affect energy resolution.

The primary cause of nonuniformity in a scintillation camera is mispositioning of individual events. Because eventpositioning is determined by the properties of the NaI(Tl) detector and the positioning electronics, changes in the range of energies of the incoming photons (i.e., scatter reduction) do not have a significant effect on field uniformity, except when very narrow (e.g., 5%) windows are used.

REFERENCE

1. Sorenson JA, Phelps ME. *Physics in Nuclear Medicine.* 2nd ed. Orlando: Grune and Stratton, 1987.

ITEM 5: COUNT RATE PERFORMANCE

Answer: *D*

A number of different techniques are used in state-of-the-art cameras to improve count rate performance. All scintillation cameras incorporate derandomizer buffers. These circuits "hold" a voltage pulse in an analog buffer until the next component in the processing circuit is ready to receive it. Because of the random nature of radioactive decay, the end result is an improved ability to count higher levels of radioactivity.

The use of dual integrator circuits also improves count rate performance. After the position of an acceptable event is determined, time is required to transfer this information to a computer or display system. By having a second parallel path, the coordinates of the first event can be transferred to the computer or display system while a second event is analyzed to determine its position. Completion of the transfer then opens the first pathway for analyzing an event while the second is transferred, etc.

In addition, it is possible to shorten the apparent dead time by shortening the integration time for the signals coming from the PMTs. However, this operation means that less light is collected from the crystal and that there is greater uncertainty in the location of individual events. The loss of spatial resolution is acceptable when higher count levels are needed for dynamic studies, such as a first-pass measurement of cardiac function.

Most cameras also incorporate pileup rejection circuits. These circuits discard pairs of events that are so close to one another in time that they distort pulse height. By rejecting these events at an early stage, less time is wasted in processing events that will have a degrading effect on the final image.

Energy-weighted acquisition (EWA) is used to improve contrast by deconvolution. As such, it has no direct effect on count rate performance. However, in the commercial system that currently offers EWA as an option, count rate performance deteriorates when both normal and EWA images are formed simultaneously.

REFERENCES

1. Sorenson JA, Phelps ME. *Physics in Nuclear Medicine.* 2nd ed. Orlando: Grune and Stratton, 1987.
2. Graham LS. Clinically applicable modifications of Anger camera technology. In: Freeman LM, Weissmann HS, eds. *Nuclear Medicine Annual 1983.* New York: Raven Press, 1983:51–96.
3. Real Time Energy Dependent Finite Spatial Filtering: WAM Brochure #A91004-M2310-M008-01-4A00. Des Plaines, Illinois: Siemens Medical Systems, Inc.
4. Breen SL, Blais M, Cradduck TD. Count rate losses under energy-weighted acquisition. *Eur J Nucl Med* 1990;16 Suppl:S82.

ITEM 6: MULTIPLE-WINDOW SPATIAL REGISTRATION ERRORS

Answer: *C*

All cameras that have more than one pulse height analyzer window incorporate special circuits to eliminate energy registration errors. Incorrect operation of these circuits may produce gain or offset errors, or both. When the image formed by photons accepted by one pulse height analyzer is a different size than that formed by photons from a second pulse height analyzer, or is offset, both spatial resolution and contrast are lost. However, this condition has no significant effect on spatial distortion, energy resolution, or resolving time.

REFERENCES

1. Graham LS. Quality assurance procedures. In: Simmons GH, ed. *The Scintillation Camera.* New York: Society of Nuclear Medicine, 1988:79–98.
2. Chapman DR, Garcia EV, Waxman AD. Misalignment of multiple photopeak analyzer outputs: effects on imaging. *J Nucl Med* 1980;21:872–874.

ITEM 7: NONCIRCULAR ORBITS

Answer: *A*

The primary problem with circular orbits in rotating single-photon emission computed tomographic (SPECT) systems lies in the fact that the scintillation camera may be at quite some distance from the body surface during some portions of the rotation arc. For example, in liver imaging the orbit must be adjusted to clear the lateral sides of the body; in the anterior position for the same radius, the camera may be as much as 10 or 12 cm from the body.

Spatial resolution degrades rapidly as a function of distance from the surface of a parallel-hole collimator. Therefore, it is important that the camera detector be at all times as close as possible to the organ of interest. This is achieved with a noncircular orbit in which either the camera head moves in and out or laterally, or the patient's bed moves so as to keep the detector surface close to the body surface at all times. A variety of mechanical motions have been implemented by different manufacturers, all with the purpose of minimizing collimator–body distance.

REFERENCE

1. Gottschalk SC, Salem D, Lim CB, et al. SPECT resolution and uniformity improvements by noncircular orbit. *J Nucl Med* 1983;24:822–828.

ITEM 8: CONE-BEAM SINGLE-PHOTON EMISSION COMPUTED TOMOGRAPHIC IMAGING

Answer: *D*

Cone-beam collimators are useful in imaging situations where the organ of interest is much smaller than the field-of-view of the camera, such as in imaging of the brain with a large field-of-view detector. By focusing the holes of the collimator in all directions, a larger fraction of the crystal surface can be used for imaging, thus allowing improved sensitivity. A cone-beam collimator can also be designed to trade off this improved sensitivity for better spatial resolution.

Although parallel-hole and fan-beam collimators generate parallel projection planes and can therefore use a two-dimensional reconstruction algorithm, cone-beam collimators generate projections that cannot be separated mathematically, and a fully three-dimensional reconstruction algorithm must be used. This results in the requirement for a more powerful array processor or, alternatively, in longer reconstruction times.

REFERENCE

1. Sorenson JA, Phelps ME. *Physics in Nuclear Medicine.* 2nd ed. Orlando: Grune and Stratton, Inc, 1987.

ITEM 9. QUALITY ASSURANCE TESTS

Answer: *C*

When major software modifications are made to the computer system by service personnel, the most prudent thing to do is to immediately back up the software before beginning any sort of analysis or data acquisition. The reason for doing this is twofold: (1) New software may contain new features that if used improperly, might result in loss of data or programs; and (2) if part of the computer fails, there could be a loss of software and data. Beginning patient data collection or analyzing unprocessed data without first performing the backup operation is risky. After the backup operation has been completed, the technologist should perform routine quality assurance (QA) procedures that involve both camera and computer. These tests should be done to ensure that the system is still capable of functioning as it was before the software upgrade. Also, it is necessary to verify that the repaired camera interface is operating properly and is adjusted for the particular camera. Without a QA test and comparison with previous QA records, the user could miss subtle problems that would have an impact on clinical operations. It is not usually necessary to perform extensive comparisons with a "gold standard" examination. Such validation studies are reserved for testing new software and equipment. However, it would be useful to reprocess some old studies whose results have been verified in order to ensure that the same results are obtained.

ITEM 10: IMAGE ARTIFACTS

Answer: *D*

An unexpected drop in recorded counts in a sharply defined area within a high-count region is most likely to be due to an overflow error. When the computer hardware fails, the data associated with a study are often lost completely. In those situations where the disks or memory fails but the computer continues to run, the images can show random loss of data or loss of an entire part of an image. Memory errors can also show individual pixels set at a value very different from surrounding pixels. Software errors generally produce error messages. When error messages are not produced but the image is changed, the results often are unexpected modifications to the entire image. Analysis of effective renal plasma flow data involves selection of regions-of-interest (ROIs) and analysis of time–activity curves. Such analysis operations would not account for the artifact described.

ITEM 11: MULTIPLE-WINDOW SPATIAL REGISTRATION ERROR

Answer: *D*

Figure 1 is an example of a marked multiple-window spatial registration error in a gallium-67 image of the right arm. Careful examination of the image at the edge of the field will show three different borders, a clear indication of an energy registration error. Because of incorrect calibration of the electronic circuits, each pulse height analyzer window of the three peaks (93, 185, and 300 keV) produces an image of a different size. The final result is an image with reduced contrast.

Analog-to-digital converter (ADC) artifacts are often associated with intensity changes along the X or Y axis, or both. Patient movement or septal penetration associated with using a low-energy collimator for high-energy photons would produce a loss of spatial resolution but could not produce the distinct borders seen in this image. The same statement can be made concerning noise in an electronic formatter.

ITEMS 12–16: SURVEY AND COUNTING INSTRUMENTS

Answers: 12, *D*; 13, *B*; 14, *C*; 15, *C*; 16, *A*

The G-M survey meter, ionization chamber survey meter, and radionuclide (dose) calibrator use gas-filled detectors operating in regions of the gas-filled detector characteristic curve that do not provide the ability to discriminate between the gamma rays emitted by indium-111 and technetium-99m.

Both NaI(Tl) and semiconductor detector systems can be used to count indium-111 in the presence of technetium-99m. The NaI(Tl) systems offer excellent detection efficiency and moderately good energy resolution (i.e., the ability to separate two gamma rays of different energies). Semiconductor detector systems provide excellent energy resolution but poor detection efficiency compared with NaI(Tl) systems. Additionally, semiconductor detector systems are more expensive to purchase, and they require either liquid nitrogen or a thermoelectric cooler to keep them at the low temperatures necessary to achieve their superior energy resolution. The NaI(Tl) systems, however, are inexpensive and require no special refrigeration.

The NaI(Tl) counting system would be preferred for the counting of a blood sample containing indium-111 and technetium-99m because detection efficiency is more important than energy resolution. The gamma rays of indium-111 are emitted at 171 and 245 keV, whereas the gamma rays from technetium-99m appear at 140 keV. The NaI(Tl) system can easily distinguish between these three gamma-ray energies. Thus, the less expensive, more readily available NaI(Tl) counting system would accomplish the task at a lower cost than the high-purity germanium semiconductor system.

The radionuclide calibrator and the NaI(Tl) and semiconductor detector systems are heavy and bulky and are designed for stationary counting of in vitro samples. Measurement of exposure rates inside a waste storage area clearly calls for a portable survey meter.

Geiger-Müller survey meters are best suited for detection of radioactive contamination and for estimation of the count rate near a low-level source of radioactivity, such as a shielded technetium generator or the hallway outside a radioactive waste storage area. Because exposure is defined only for air, and G-M detectors contain organically-based gases, a G-M survey meter cannot measure exposure or exposure rate. The scale of a G-M survey meter *can* be cross-calibrated to give an exposure reading if the radionuclide used for calibration is the same radionuclide being measured clinically; this type of cross-calibration is extremely difficult and is almost never done.

The ionization chamber survey meter uses a detector that is filled with air, so it can measure exposure directly. Additionally, ionization chamber survey meters measure the currents created by the many ion pairs created within the chamber rather than the individual pulses detected by the G-M detector, so ionization chamber survey meters can be used for much more intense radiation fields. For example, the radiation output of a linear accelerator used in a radiation therapy clinic is measured with ionization chambers. Exposure rates from urine containing iodine-131 after iodine-131 therapy for thyroid cancer may be assumed to be quite high because patients with thyroid carcinoma are typically treated with 3,700 MBq or more, and their urine may contain 85% or more of the administered activity. Therefore, the ionization chamber survey meter would be preferred because it measures exposure rate directly, and it does not have the dead-time losses that might cause the G-M survey meter to give erroneously low readings in such a high radiation field.

The survey meters measure exposure or count rates, and the NaI(Tl) and semiconductor detector systems count individual gamma-ray events. None of these systems measures activity directly. With proper calibration and careful performance of measurements, computers associated with NaI(Tl) and semiconductor detector systems could calculate the activity of a sample and display an estimated activity. Use of these systems in this manner is rare, fraught with the potential for procedural errors, and discouraged.

All the current commercial radionuclide calibrators have either hardware or software "switches" to allow the operator to display activity readings in either SI units (becquerels) or the old units (curies). Most of these instruments are autoranging and will automatically display the appropriate submultiple or supermultiple of the selected unit. Although the flexibility of switching back and forth between the two systems of units makes the calibrators more marketable worldwide, the operator must be very careful to make sure that the switch is not in the "curies" position when he or she is expecting to receive a reading in becquerels. Some calibrators allow the knob of the "units" switch to be locked into one position with a key to prevent inadvertent mispositioning. Such safeguards are less easy to implement when the units are selected by software.

Gas-filled survey meters use detectors that are usually cylindrical, pancake-shaped, or in the shape of a truncated cone. Reentrant wells are never used in gas-filled detectors for nuclear medicine applications, except for radionuclide calibrators.

Semiconductor and NaI(Tl) detector systems can be purchased with either flat-faced or reentrant-well designs. The flat-faced detectors are less expensive, but the reentrant-well detectors offer much improved geometric efficiency for only a small additional capital cost. Flat-faced NaI(Tl) detectors were very common in probe systems, such as renogram and thyroid uptake probes. Although reentrant-well NaI(Tl) detectors have been available for many years, the technology for producing semiconductor detectors has only recently advanced to where the semiconductor crystals can economically be grown sufficiently large to permit the introduction of a reentrant well.

Radionuclide calibrators have always used reentrant-well ionization chambers, whether operated with air at ambient pressure or with argon at elevated pressures. One company attempted to market an instrument that used a pancake-shaped NaI(Tl) crystal at the bottom of a sample holder, but it did not work well and failed soon after introduction.

Ionization chamber survey meters and radionuclide calibrators use ionization chambers operating in the current mode, that is, the number of ion pairs being created per second is so large that the net effect of all of the ion pairs is detected rather than the pulses corresponding to each individual ion pair. Because dead time is defined as the time that must elapse after the first event before the next event can be detected, and because individual events are not detected in these instruments, ionization chamber survey meters and radionuclide calibrators do not exhibit dead time.

Semiconductor detector and NaI(Tl) systems detect individual gamma rays and exhibit measurable but comparably short dead times (on the order of 1 μsec or less). Count rates can be on the order of hundreds of thousands of counts per second with these systems.

The dead time of a G-M detector can be on the order of hundreds of microseconds, which restricts the useful count rate to a few tens of thousands of counts per second. The dead time is very large because each ion pair that creates a pulse causes the detector to completely discharge, and the approximately 900-V potential difference is restored by recharging a circuit element of large capacitance and, therefore, long charging time. The G-M detector on most nuclear medicine survey meters is relatively large and is designed for use in radiation fields of 100 mR/hr or less. Special G-M survey meters can be purchased that have a small, lower dead-time internal G-M detector that allows them to be used in radiation fields of about 1 R/hr. The meter usually does not remind the user that it has switched to the internal detector when the radiation fields are high, so operators must exercise care to avoid misusing these types of meters.

ITEMS 17–21: QUALITY CONTROL FOR SCINTILLATION CAMERAS

Answers: 17, *A*; 18, *B*; 19, *D*; 20, *D*; 21, *D*

It is generally recommended that field uniformity tests be performed each day that a scintillation camera is used. This includes weekends and holidays on which emergency procedures must be performed. Linearity (distortion) can be evaluated from images of a resolution test pattern that is normally checked once a week. Areas of significant nonlinearity can usually be matched with the nonuniformity visualized in the flood field images.

The maximum count rate must be tested on a periodic basis. Drift of electronic components may produce a loss of count rate performance and an increase in resolving time. There is no consensus with regard to the frequency for this test, but it is reasonable to perform this measurement each quarter, in compliance with recent requirements of the Joint Commission for Accreditation of Healthcare Organizations (JCAHO) for quarterly performance tests.

Consensus is also lacking with regard to the recommended frequency for measuring sensitivity and multiple-window spatial registration. However, it is reasonable to apply the same logic as for measuring the maximum count rate, that is, these tests should be performed each quarter.

REFERENCE

1. Graham LS. Quality assurance procedures. In: Simmons GH, ed. The Scintillation Camera. New York: Society of Nuclear Medicine, 1988:79–98.

ITEMS 22–26: FLOOD FIELD NONUNIFORMITY

Answers: 22, *C*; 23, *B*; 24, *A*; 25, *D*; 26, *E*

The image in Figure 2A shows a focal defect due to a cracked crystal. Slight edge packing (increased intensity around the edge) can be seen in the flood field image. A similar defect could be produced by a damaged collimator, but a damaged collimator would not produce edge packing.

The image presented in Figure 2B was taken with a pulse height analyzer window set on the high side of the photopeak. Even though the tubes are clearly visualized as hot spots, the pattern is essentially symmetric for a properly tuned camera.

A poorly tuned camera may present an image such as that shown in Figure 2C. Both hot and cold spots can be visualized. In contrast to the image presented in Figure 2B, there is a lack of symmetry in the tube pattern.

The bone scan shown in Figure 2D contains an ADC artifact. It appears as a faint vertical, linear defect on the right side of the image (patient's left side), approximately halfway between the center and the edge of the image. At that location, events are positioned improperly. The appearance of the artifact (linear) and its direction (vertical) suggests a problem with the ADC that digitizes signals in the X direction, as was the case. A defective collimator might produce a similar image. A flood image taken without the collimator in place would reveal the true cause.

One of the problems associated with the use of a liquid-filled technetium-99m flood source is failure to thoroughly mix the solution. This is shown in Figure 2E. Such a flood source should not be used to check field uniformity because detector nonuniformities would be difficult to identify. Neither should such a source be used to acquire high-count floods for flood-correcting single-photon emission computed tomographic (SPECT) studies because it would produce significant artifacts in the reconstructed images.

ITEMS 27–29: POSITRON EMISSION TOMOGRAPHIC AND SINGLE-PHOTON EMISSION COMPUTED TOMOGRAPHIC CHARACTERISTICS

Answers: 27, *C*; 28, *B*; 29, *B*

Any method that reconstructs transverse sections using computed tomographic (CT) principles (SPECT, positron emission tomography [PET]) will enhance contrast relative to a planar technique that superimposes overlying and underlying structures. In general, PET imaging is considered to be quantitatively more accurate than SPECT imaging. This is in part due to the fact that in PET imaging, the attenuation is independent of the depth at which the positron annihilation takes place. It is customary in PET imaging to perform a transmission scan, particularly in imaging the heart, thereby further improving the quantitative accuracy.

However, the emphasis in PET imaging on accurate quantitation is largely because PET is most often used in research. Transmission imaging is certainly possible in SPECT and can be used to improve the quantitative accuracy of SPECT attenuation correction.

ITEMS 30–33: BASIC PROPERTIES OF VARIOUS SINGLE-PHOTON EMISSION COMPUTED TOMOGRAPHIC SCANNERS

Answers: 30, *A*; 31, *D*; 32, *D*; 33, *E*

Dedicated SPECT scanners using an annular crystal have the advantage that the detector assembly can be kept stationary, and only the collimator rotates. Such scanners are best suited for brain imaging because the brain is completely surrounded by the detector, and the detector is quite close to the brain, thereby optimizing spatial resolution. Conversely, this geometry has the disadvantage that the detector radius is fixed. Although it is possible to conceive of an annular crystal scanner for the body, such a device would not be optimal for brain imaging because the detectors would be too far from the organ of interest.

Rotating Anger cameras with one to four detectors can be used for brain imaging (fan-beam collimators improve the performance of brain imaging) and can equally well be used for body imaging provided that the radius of rotation of the detectors is variable.

ITEMS 34–37: COMPUTER MEMORY AND STORAGE

Answers: 34, *B*; 35, *C*; 36, *A*; 37, *D*

Gated cardiac studies require rapid acquisition of a large amount of data into preallocated frames in memory. When more memory is available, more images can be stored, which provides improved temporal resolution. Cache memory, a special type of high-speed memory that is available in some computers, can be used in the collection and processing of a gated cardiac study. However, cache memory is limited in size and is designed specifically to speed up access to data by the central processing unit (CPU) from disk or main memory. This speed is seen as an overall improvement in performance of the system in comparison with a system not having cache memory. Cache memory is not used for general-purpose data storage.

Optical disk storage is an excellent storage medium for archival purposes (write once, read many times) or for intermediate storage (read/write disk) but is far too slow to support the multiframe image acquisition required for gated cardiac studies. The same problems associated with optical disks are also associated with hard disks. Hard disks can store a gated study after it is collected or can be used for nonframe mode (list mode or gated list mode) acquisition. Floppy disks have neither the capacity nor the speed to permit gated studies to be stored on them during collection.

A day's worth of clinical studies could consist of several examinations that are collections of different types of studies. All data for the day must be stored until the attending physicians can read the images. Maintaining enough random-access memory to store these studies is too expensive to be practical. An optical disk is usually used as a long-term archival storage medium because of its large capacity and write once, read many times technology. Hard disks are relatively inexpensive, can hold large amounts of data, are read/write media that are randomly accessible, and are ideal for intermediate storage. Depending on the size of the hard disk, several day's worth of images can be stored before the data are archived to optical disk or magnetic tape. Several floppy disks could be used to store a day's studies, but data transfer would be very slow.

Large numbers of images can be archived in several ways. Sometimes it is practical to store images for a long time on a hard disk, but this approach can be expensive. Sometimes it is practical to store a large number of images in small groups on a large number of floppy disks, but storage room can be a problem. Memory of any type is not useful for long-term storage because of the size, cost, and volatility of semiconductor memory. An ideal archival medium is the optical disk. Because an optical disk can hold as much as 1–2 gigabytes, over 250,000 images ($64 \times 64 \times 1$ byte) can be stored. This may represent several years' worth of information for a medium-sized nuclear medicine department. Coupled with the high storage density of optical disks, they have a projected lifetime of 30 years.

REFERENCES

1. Erickson JJ. Nuclear medicine computer hardware. In: Erickson JJ, Rollo FD, eds. *Digital Nuclear Medicine.* Philadelphia: JB Lippincott, 1983:47–59.
2. Simmons GH, Kereiakes JG, Pickens DR, Erickson JJ. Computer hardware and software fundamentals. *Radiographics* 1985;5:11–30.

ITEMS 38–42: TYPES OF DATA ACQUISITION

Answers: 38, *B*; 39, *D*; 40, *C*; 41, *A*; 42, *B*

There are a number of different ways to collect the data in a nuclear medicine environment. Proper selection of a data collection protocol depends on the type of study that is to be performed. For a first-pass cardiac study, the goal is to acquire data as rapidly as possible during the passage of the radiopharmaceutical through the heart. This will usually require a list mode acquisition to handle the high data rates that are likely to be present. Gating information is usually recorded as well so that several cardiac cycles can be used to track the bolus of activity through the heart. Images are created after collection by reframing the data. Ventriculograms at rest are usually collected by using conventional gated acquisition. The data rates expected are easily accommodated by nuclear medicine computers so that the images can be built up in memory over multiple cardiac cycles. Renal function studies can be collected with a conventional dynamic acquisition, where there is no need for physiological gating. Images are collected at a specified frame rate for a specified time. Planar liver imaging is usually performed as a static imaging study, requiring that the computer produce an image that is the result of a specified number of counts or length of time. Cardiac studies in the presence of arrhythmias are most readily accommodated by gated list mode acquisitions because data associated with irregular periods can be ignored during the subsequent reframing process.

REFERENCES

1. Gelfand MJ, Thomas SR, eds. *Effective Use of Computers in Nuclear Medicine.* New York: McGraw-Hill, 1988.
2. Jones JP. Nuclear medicine operating systems. In: Erickson JJ, Rollo FD, eds. *Digital Nuclear Medicine.* Philadelphia: JB Lippincott, 1983:105–154.

ITEMS 43–47: IMAGE PROCESSING

Answers: 43, *D*; 44, *D*; 45, *C*; 46, *A*; 47, *B*

Phase analysis is a technique that is used to perform functional analysis of gated cardiac studies. It is based on computing one or more harmonics (sinusoidal components) of the time–activity curve for each pixel in the images from a study. This analysis method creates one phase and one amplitude image from the series of gated images. Thus, phase analysis provides color-coded functional images representing the extent of motion and the time of onset of motion for each portion of the heart.

In the analysis of a series of rapid-sequence images, the desired output is a time–activity curve representing the movement of an isotope through the target organ. Many analysis programs will request that the user mark on one image the boundaries of an ROI that will be used throughout an image set. An edge detector will then be used to select the region on each successive slice automatically. The edge detector is usually able to follow the changing size of an organ, such as the left ventricle, to produce an ROI from the computer-generated time–activity curve.

In dynamic studies, a bolus of radioisotope-labelled material is injected into a peripheral vein. By the time the bolus arrives at the target organ, it has usually passed through the lungs, heart and other vascular structures and is spread out significantly. As a result, the time–activity curve from a region-of-interest set over the organ of interest does not accurately represent the temporal passage of radioactivity through the vasculature. Deconvolution is a mathematical technique by which the broadening of a time–activity curve is corrected for the shape of the input function (bolus).

Noise in an image can reduce the effectiveness of ROI analysis methods as well as obscure details that may be of clinical significance. Noise can usually be reduced by filtering an image. Filters can be designed that are very simple, such as nine-point smoothing filters, or can be much more complex, such as Butterworth bandpass filters, which require the use of Fourier transformation to implement.

Back projection is an image reconstruction method that permits planar images from a SPECT data collection set to be formed into tomographic images.

REFERENCES

1. Gelfand MJ, Thomas SR, eds. *Effective Use of Computers in Nuclear Medicine.* New York: McGraw-Hill, 1988.
2. Jones JP. Clinical imaging studies. In: Erickson JJ, Rollo FD, eds. *Digital Nuclear Medicine.* Philadelphia: JB Lippincott, 1983:105–154.
3. Garcia EV, Train KV, Maddahi J, et al. Quantification of rotational thallium-201 myocardial tomography. *J Nucl Med* 1985;26:17–26.
4. Byron E, Pavel DG, Swiryn S, Mayer-Pavel C. Phase images of gated cardiac studies: a standard evaluation procedure. In: Esser PD, ed. *Functional Mapping of Organ Systems.* New York: Society of Nuclear Medicine, 1982:129.

ITEMS 48–52: DOSE CALIBRATORS

Answers: 48, *T*; 49, *T*; 50, *F*; 51, *T*; 52, *F*

Radionuclide calibrators have been manufactured with reentrant-well ionization chambers that operate either with air at ambient temperature and pressure or with argon at about 12 atm. Regardless of the pressure, both of these types of chambers are relatively inefficient for the detection of gamma rays because the absorption coefficients for air and argon are very small, and the dimensions of the chambers are also small. If the same radioactive sample were placed in two chambers of the same size and shape with one containing ambient air or pressurized argon, the chamber containing the pressurized argon would produce a larger electrical current from the increased number of ion pairs caused by the higher absorption coefficient. If the activity of the sample were low, the ambient air chamber might give off a very weak signal that would be difficult to distinguish from electronic noise, whereas the pressurized argon chamber would display a stronger signal easily distinguished from noise. The pressurized argon chamber would therefore exhibit a higher sensitivity at low activity levels.

The reentrant-well design optimizes geometric efficiency by surrounding the sample almost completely with the detector. When the sample is placed in the bottom of the well, only a small fraction of the gamma rays emitted from the sample can escape from the well without passing through the detector gas. As the sample is raised toward the top of the well, either by physically lifting it or by increasing the volume in which the activity is diluted, the fraction of gamma rays that can escape through the open mouth of the well increases, and the efficiency of the detector decreases. Additionally, as the sample moves toward the mouth of the well, the path length of the gamma rays in the counting gas inside the detector decreases, and there is less likelihood of interaction. The decreased path length is of greater importance in the ambient air chamber because of the lower absorption coefficient, that is, the total electrical current induced in the chamber decreases, and the indicated activity is falsely low. The pressurized argon chamber suffers from decreased path length as well, but the significantly higher absorption coefficient causes the loss of current to be smaller and the inaccuracy in the activity reading to be less. Thus, the ambient air chamber exhibits greater variability in its accuracy when samples are of different geometries (e.g., 1-ml syringe versus 30-ml glass vial) and different volumes (e.g., 1-ml syringe versus 60-ml syringe).

The effect of a high room background, due to inadequate shielding of a technetium generator, is to generate a small electrical current in the detector even when no sample is placed in the well. High room background has the same effect as excessive electronic noise, that is, the strength of the electrical current caused by a radioactive sample placed in the well must be large enough to be reliably detected above the "noise." In other words, the signal must be sufficiently large for the signal-to-noise ratio to be statistically significant. The signal is made larger by increasing the activity of the sample. If the activity of the sample must be increased to overcome the high room background, then the inherent advantage of the pressurized argon chamber at low activities is lost, and its accuracy becomes comparable to that of the ambient air chamber.

ITEMS 53–57: THALLIUM-DOPED SODIUM IODIDE WELL DETECTORS

Answers: 53, *F*; 54, *T*; 55, *T*; 56, *T*; 57, *F*

The NaI(Tl) crystal produces tiny scintillations of light when ionizing radiation strikes it. These scintillations would be almost impossible to detect with the human eye, so they are transformed into electrons by the photocathode of a PMT and amplified by the PMT to produce a pulse that is large enough to be handled with relatively simple electronics. Any light that strikes the photocathode of the PMT will cause electrons to be emitted and a pulse to be generated; it is therefore critical for low-activity performance that all stray light be excluded. Most modern NaI(Tl) well detectors are purchased from the manufacturer encased in an aluminum can that completely encloses the NaI(Tl) crystal and the PMT in a light-tight environment. Lead is not used for the case because it would prevent low-energy gamma rays from penetrating the NaI(Tl) crystal.

NaI(Tl) is hygroscopic (i.e., it readily absorbs water). If NaI(Tl) absorbs water, it turns yellow and cannot efficiently transfer the scintillations to the PMT photocathode, resulting in decreased response and falsely low readings. Thus, NaI(Tl) crystals are carefully packaged with hermetic seals to prevent the entry of moisture.

The wells of the radionuclide dose calibrator and the NaI(Tl) well counter are sufficiently deep to maximize geometric efficiency, that is, they allow very few gamma rays to escape without interacting within the surrounding detector. If a sample were completely surrounded by detector, such as in liquid scintillation counting, we would say that 4π geometry exists. The NaI(Tl) well counter is as close as we can come to 4π geometry within the cost constraints of growing large NaI(Tl) crystals.

When a gamma ray interacts in a NaI(Tl) crystal, the emission of light occurs rapidly, as does the amplification of the signal by the PMT. In fact, the pulse emitted by the PMT is so sharp and narrow that conventional, inexpensive amplifiers and pulse height analyzers would have great difficulty handling the rapid change in voltage. A preamplifier accepts the sharp, narrow PMT pulse as input and converts it to a broader pulse that is better suited to the amplifier and pulse height analyzer. All NaI(Tl) detector systems use a preamplifier between the PMT and the amplifier.

ITEMS 58–61: RADIONUCLIDE CALIBRATOR CONSTANCY TESTS

Answers: 58, *T*; 59, *T*; 60, *F*; 61, *T*

The electrical currents generated in the ionization chamber of a radionuclide calibrator are very small and require sophisticated electronics to amplify and analyze them. These electronics are prone to drift over time and must be tested frequently enough to detect and correct large changes in detector performance. Radionuclide calibrator constancy checks must be performed each day of use, before the first clinical usage. Because the circuit that transforms ionization chamber current into activity is simply a digital voltmeter, it makes no difference what radionuclide is used, and only a single standard needs to be measured. The most commonly used radionuclides are cesium-137 and cobalt-57. Cesium-137 has a 30-year half-life, which means that radioactive decay corrections of source activity do not have to be performed every day, and the source itself does not have to be replaced very often. The disadvantage of cesium-137 is that its gamma ray is emitted at 662 keV, which is much higher than any clinically used gamma rays. Cobalt-57, conversely, emits 122-keV gamma rays that closely approximate those of technetium-99m and other clinically important radionuclides. Cobalt-57 sources are usually manufactured with activities of 3–10 mCi, activities that are representative of clinical dosages. The disadvantages of cobalt-57 are its high cost and its 270-day halflife, which necessitates frequent decay correction and frequent source replacement.

At the time of an annual calibration, a radionuclide dose calibrator must be able to measure activities to within ±5%. In daily usage, it must be able to measure clinical activities to within ±10%. If the constancy check exhibits a variation from the known activity of the check source of more than 10% (in either direction), the cause of the variation must be ascertained and corrected before the calibrator can be used for clinical samples.

ITEMS 62–66: LIQUID SCINTILLATION COUNTERS

Answers: 62, *T*; 63, *T*; 64, *F*; 65, *T*; 66, *F*

Liquid scintillation counters were developed for the counting of weakly penetrating radiations, such as beta particles and very low energy x- and gamma rays. Common radionuclides assayed by liquid scintillation counting include hydrogen-3 (tritium), carbon-14, phosphorus-32, sulfur-35, and iodine-125. In liquid scintillation counting, the radioactive sample is dissolved or dispersed as uniformly as possible in the counting fluid. Gels are sometimes used to achieve uniform dispersions when the sample is particulate or particularly immiscible in the counting fluid. Counting fluids were originally composed primarily of organic solvents, which caused problems when water-based samples were counted. These organic solvents were also hazardous and required special handling for disposal. Recently, water-based counting fluids have been introduced. These new fluids, or "cocktails," can be used with water-based samples and can be discarded through the sanitary sewer system if the radioactivity levels are low enough.

Water, oxygen, and a number of common biochemical substances (e.g., hemoglobin, urea, chlorophyll) interfere with the transfer of radiation energy from the sample into scintillations and ultimately into electronic pulses in the PMT; this interference is called quenching. Quench correction factors are vitally important to the accurate counting of liquid scintillation samples and are performed automatically by all modern counting systems. Each manufacturer uses a proprietary method for quench correction, but in general these methods compare the level of quenching in the sample being counted with a quench correction curve derived from a series of samples with known quenching.

When liquid scintillation counters were first developed, PMTs operated at room temperature exhibited very high electronic noise (so-called dark current). This high noise level was caused by the ease with which electrons spontaneously were ejected from the photocathode and the dynodes. At that time, the only way to reduce the dark current was to operate the PMT at refrigerator or freezer temperatures, and the earliest liquid scintillation counters were frequently chest-type freezers with the sample holder and PMTs mounted on the floor of the freezer compartment. As photocathode research produced "quieter" materials, the need to refrigerate the PMTs gradually disappeared. Modern liquid scintillation counters can be purchased with refrigeration systems, but the refrigeration is designed for special sample handling requirements rather than for PMT considerations. Some liquid scintillation counters can be purchased with heaters that allow operation at elevated temperatures.

ITEMS 67–71: MULTICHANNEL ANALYZERS

Answers: 67, *T*; 68, *F*; 69, *T*; 70, *F*; 71, *F*

When a 1000-channel multichannel analyzer (MCA) is calibrated for 1000-keV full scale, each channel represents 1 keV (e.g., the 140-keV gamma ray from technetium-99m would appear in channel 140). Although the energy calibration (kiloelectron volt per channel) could be verified using any radionuclide with a known gamma-ray energy, cesium-137 is preferred because of its usefulness for other required checks. The cesium-137 rod source is placed in the well, and the cesium-137 window is displayed on the cathode ray tube (CRT) monitor. The 662-keV gamma-ray photopeak from cesium-137 should appear in channel 662. If it does not, the amplifier gain is used to slide the photopeak up or down until it is in the correct channel. For this test, the activity of the rod source is not important so long as it is low enough to avoid dead-time losses. Thus, it is not necessary to decay correct the source activity on a daily basis to check channel energy calibration.

The NaI(Tl) detector systems contain many components that are subject to electronic drift, which can evidence itself as incorrect channel energy calibration and as reduced counting efficiency. A daily constancy check must be performed to ensure that significant drift in efficiency has not occurred. A cesium-137 rod source is usually used for the daily constancy check because it has a long half-life that obviates the need for frequent decay correction and because the cesium-137 source is already being used for the channel energy calibration check. A common procedure is to check the channel energy calibration and then to immediately count the source for 1 min with the verified window placement. The counts in the cesium-137 window are then plotted on a quality control graph or entered into a logbook and compared with the expected reading.

The downscatter of the 364-keV gamma rays of iodine-131 into the 140-keV window of technetium-99m occurs regardless of the resolution of the MCA and cannot be ignored. Semiconductor detectors cause less of a Compton plateau than NaI(Tl), but even semiconductor detector systems must take downscatter into account when attempting to quantitate technetium-99m in the presence of iodine-131.

If the NaI(Tl) well has become contaminated with iodine-131, a background count would exhibit counts in the iodine-131 window; similarly, technetium-99m contamination would appear in the technetium-99m window. The cesium-137 window is centered on 662 keV and is usually roughly 100 keV wide. It is very unlikely that low-level contamination by iodine-131 or technetium-99m would be detected in the cesium-137 window. Even high-level contamination might be missed if only the cesium-137 window was checked, because summing of technetium-99m and iodine-131 gamma rays would create a sum peak below the bottom of the cesium-137 window (504 versus 612 keV, respectively). A better check for contamination would be to set a 0–1,000-keV window and to visually inspect the background spectrum for unanticipated peaks.

ITEMS 72–76: THALLIUM-DOPED SODIUM IODIDE WELL COUNTERS

Answers: 72, *T*; 73, *F*; 74, *T*; 75, *F*; 76, *F*

As a rough approximation, assume that the blood volume of the patient was 5,000 ml, so that the concentration of technetium-99m in the blood samples was 0.1 MBq/ml (500 MBq/5,000 ml) or less. Significant dead-time losses can occur whenever the activity in the well of a NaI(Tl) detector exceeds 0.04 MBq (1 μCi), so at least some of the blood samples collected during this study will be too radioactive to count inside the well. A 2-hr delay before counting will reduce the activity in each sample to 79% of the original value, a value that will still be at least twice the desirable level for the hottest samples. The samples can be counted immediately at the end of the collection period if the samples are suspended in a reproducible geometry (position) above the detector rather than in the well. The resultant degradation of geometric efficiency will reduce the dead-time losses to acceptable levels. Decreasing the width of the window will not affect dead-time losses because every pulse must be fully analyzed before being placed into its proper MCA channel regardless of whether it will ultimately fall within the window. In fact, in MCAs, windows are a postacquisition form of data processing, and they have no influence on the speed of data acquisition.

A 7-ml tube filled with blood will have a significant portion of its length protruding from the top of the well. The fraction of the contents that is outside the well will be detected with relatively poor efficiency compared with that inside the well. If the serum and solid fractions of the blood are homogeneously mixed, the technetium-99m–containing serum will be present throughout the length of the tube and will yield a count rate that is a combination of the efficiencies inside and outside the well. If the tube is counted on the next day, with the red cell layer on the bottom and serum layer on the top, the count rate will be much lower (even after decay correction) because most of the serum will now be positioned outside the well, and the efficiency of counting will be much poorer.

The geometric efficiency of a well detector is best when the sample is very small and located in the bottom of the well. If the concentration of radioactivity in a sample is kept constant but the volume is increased, the count rate is seen to increase at a less than linear rate. The incremental volumes that are added are closer and closer to the exit port of the well and therefore undergo decreasing geometric efficiency. The preferable solution in this instance would be to reduce all serum samples to 1 ml and count the samples for a longer period of time.

ITEMS 77–81: UNIFORMITY CORRECTION DEVICES IN SCINTILLATION CAMERAS

Answers: 77, *F*; 78, *F*; 79, *T*; 80, *T*; 81, *F*

Count skimming, count addition, and unblank modulation do not correct for the fundamental causes of nonuniformity in a scintillation camera. They simply remove counts from "hot" areas, add counts to "cool" areas, or leave the dot on the CRT for a longer time in "cool" areas. All these operations are based on a flood field reference image that is stored in microprocessor memory on a regular basis. Although these operations produce a cosmetically uniformly corrected flood field image, they do not correct for the fundamental causes of nonuniformity, namely, shifts of the photopeak and the incorrect positioning of individual events. In clinical studies these errors may produce a reduction in the accuracy of quantitative procedures. Distortion correction circuits use carefully prepared "maps" of nonlinearity in the detector to correct in live time for errors in the positioning of individual events. In similar fashion, "maps" of the position of the photopeak are used to correct for misalignment of the photopeak with the analyzer window (energy errors). The end result is a much more accurate image of the spatial distribution and intensity of gamma ray interactions with the detector.

REFERENCES

1. Graham LS. Clinically applicable modifications of Anger camera technology. In: Freeman LM, Weissmann HS, eds. *Nuclear Medicine Annual 1983.* New York: Raven Press, 1983:51–96.
2. Busemann-Sokole E, Farrell TJ, Cradduck TD. Effect of scintillation camera nonuniformity on ejection fraction measurements. *J Nucl Med* 1985; 1323–1330.

ITEMS 82–86: INTRINSIC SPATIAL RESOLUTION

Answers: 82, *F*; 83, *T*; 84, *T*; 85, *F*; 86, *F*

In recent years there has been a significant improvement in the intrinsic (uncollimated) spatial resolution of Anger scintillation cameras, primarily due to the increased number of PMTs, which provides finer sampling of the distribution of light in the crystal. A second factor that has contributed to the improved spatial resolution is a decrease in the thickness of the light pipes or their entire removal. This alters the distribution of light as seen by the photocathodes of the PMTs. Although distortion correction circuits improve field uniformity, they produce no significant changes in spatial resolution. Shortening the time that the dot stays on the CRT *(unblank time)* does not improve spatial resolution. In fact, shortened unblank times are generally used when the time to process individual events is decreased, which actually produces a loss of spatial resolution. Less light means greater uncertainty with regard to the position of an event, hence, poorer spatial resolution.

All other factors being equal, the use of thin-walled foil collimators provide an improvement in system, but not intrinsic, spatial resolution. By definition, system spatial resolution refers to the resolution of the detector plus the collimator and may be measured without or with the presence of scatter.

REFERENCE

1. Adams R. The scintillation gamma camera. In: Williams L, ed. *Nuclear Medicine Physics.* Vol. II. Boca Raton, FL: CRC Press, 1987:89–154.

ITEMS 87–91: OFF-PEAK IMAGING

Answers: 87, *F*; 88, *F*; 89, *T*; 90, *F*; 91, *F*

The use of off-peak imaging has waxed and waned during the development of nuclear medicine. The rationale for off-peak imaging is based on the fact that Compton scattering of photons in the patient produces a loss of energy. For relatively small scattering angles (less than 55°), the loss of energy is not sufficiently great to exclude acceptance of the scattered photon by a 20% energy window. In fact, the energies of many scattered photons overlap the Gaussian distribution of perceived energies for unscattered photons interacting with the camera crystal. Because these scattered photons are on the low-energy side of the photopeak, the composite spectrum is skewed. Positioning the pulse height analyzer window asymmetrically, that is, shifting it approximately 8 keV to the high side of the technetium-99m photopeak results in a differentially greater rejection of scattered than unscattered photons. The end result is an improvement in contrast with an associated lowering of the observer count rate. This effect makes off-peak imaging undesirable for dynamic studies for which it is more important to increase the number of counts obtained per unit time than to improve image contrast.

In some cameras, particularly those that do not use a light pipe, there may be a loss of field uniformity with even relatively small shifts of the pulse height analyzer window. This would increase the possibility of producing artifacts or falsely positive image interpretations, or both.

Off-peak imaging does not improve or cause a loss of energy registration. Energy registration is lost when the circuits contained in all MCA scintillation cameras are out of calibration, and there is either an improper alignment (offset error) or difference in image size (gain error) when the images from different pulse height analyzer windows are compared.

REFERENCES

1. La Fontaine RL, Stein MA, Graham LS, et al. Cold lesions: enhanced contrast using asymmetric photopeak windows. *Radiology* 1986;60:255–260.
2. Graham LS, La Fontaine RL, Stein MA. Effects of asymmetric photopeak windows on flood field uniformity and spatial resolution of scintillation cameras. *J Nucl Med* 1986;27:706–713.
3. Collier BD, Palmer DW, Knobel J, et al. Gamma camera energy windows for Tc-99m bone scintigraphy: effect of asymmetry on contrast resolution. *Radiology* 1984;151:495–497.

ITEMS 92–95: CONVERGING COLLIMATORS

Answers: 92, *T*; 93, *F*; 94, *T*; 95, *T*

Because of the magnifying property of the converging collimator, spatial resolution at any distance is better than that of a parallel-hole collimator. In addition, spatial resolution degrades more slowly than in a parallel-hole collimator. However, this improvement in resolution comes at the expense of field-of-view, that is, the size of the area that can be imaged.

Because of the angulation of the holes there is also an increase in efficiency, and more counts will be accepted per unit time from a target that is small enough to be in the field-of-view of the collimator. These advantages are offset by one potentially serious problem. Images are distorted because the magnification changes with distance from the collimator face. Small objects that are farther away from the face may appear to be the same size as larger objects that are close to the collimator.

REFERENCES

1. Tsui BMW. Collimator design, properties, and characteristics. In: Simmons GH, ed. *The Scintillation Camera.* New York, Society of Nuclear Medicine, 1988:17–45.
2. Moyer RA. A low-energy multihole converging collimator compared with a pinhole collimator. *J Nucl Med* 1974;15:59–74.
3. Adams R. The scintillation gamma camera. In: Williams L, ed. *Nuclear Medicine Physics.* Vol II. Boca Raton, FL: CRC Press, 1987:89–154.

ITEMS 96–100: IMPROVEMENT OF IMAGE CONTRAST

Answers: 96, *T*; 97, *T*; 98, *T*; 99, *F*; 100, *F*

Several different techniques can be used to improve contrast by removing scatter from radionuclide images. Shifting the pulse height analyzer window to the high side of the photopeak will produce a disproportionately greater rejection of scattered photons than unscattered photons. Cameras with better energy resolution can determine the energy of a photon more accurately. This in turn makes possible the use of narrower pulse height analyzer windows (e.g., 15% versus 20%), which decreases the angle by which a photon can be scattered and still be accepted in the pulse height analyzer window. Widening the analyzer window increases the acceptance of scattered photons by recording as true events crystal interactions by photons that have been scattered through a greater angle. The result will be a loss of image contrast.

Energy-weighted acquisition utilizes information from scatter events to improve image contrast. Use of a low-resolution collimator will reduce spatial resolution but does not improve contrast.

REFERENCES

1. Real Time Energy Dependent Finite Spatial Filtering: WAM Brochure No. A91004-M2310-M008-01-4A00. Des Plaines, Illinois: Siemens Medical Systems, Inc.
2. La Fontaine R, Stein MA, Graham LS, et al. Cold lesions: enhanced contrast using asymmetric photopeak windows. *Radiology* 1986;160:255–260.

ITEMS 101–105: SMART CONSOLES

Answers: 101, *T*; 102, *T*; 103, *F*; 104, *F*; 105, *T*

The integration of microprocessor technology and detector electronics with modern scintillation camera design has produced a more efficient imaging unit. The microprocessor-based intelligence of many consoles provides the ability to set up protocols, compensate for different types of film, and perform simple analyses of clinical studies. However, even though energy and distortion correction also involve microprocessors, these operations are performed normally by the detector electronics.

ITEMS 106–109: POSITRON EMISSION TOMOGRAPHIC IMAGING

Answers: 106, *T*; 107, *F*; 108, *F*; 109, *T*

Positron emission tomographic imaging detects two 511-keV photons emitted in opposite directions after the annihilation of a positron and an electron. Therefore, mechanical collimation is not necessary. The elimination of the collimator allows high spatial resolution to be achieved by using a high-resolution detector without the loss in sensitivity associated with the use of a collimator. Positron emission tomographs typically achieve 5-mm spatial resolution with 5 to 20 times the sensitivity of SPECT scanners.

REFERENCE

1. Sorenson JA, Phelps ME. *Physics in Nuclear Medicine.* 2nd ed. Orlando: Grune and Stratton, 1987.

ITEMS 110–113: CHARACTERISTICS OF SINGLE-PHOTON EMISSION COMPUTED TOMOGRAPHY IMAGING

Answers: 110, *F*; 111, *T*; 112, *T*; 113, *F*

Rotating Anger camera SPECT systems have the best spatial resolution at all points that are close to the collimator surface, (i.e., at the periphery of the reconstructed image). Because the patient is imaged from all sides, spatial resolution is relatively uniform but degrades somewhat toward the center of the field-of-view in the transverse plane.

A planar image is a projection image in which all activity at right angles to the collimator is superimposed. This superposition reduces the contrast of individual structures. Reconstruction of the full three-dimensional distribution restores the initial high contrast. Because rotating Anger camera SPECT systems provide multiple slices in which the thickness of the slice is the same as the X and Y dimensions of the pixels in individual transverse sections (provided pixel size calibrations are current), sagittal and coronal views can be displayed without the acquisition of additional data.

Quality control is extremely important for high-quality artifact-free images. Not only must the camera itself have good spatial resolution and uniformity, but in addition, the center of rotation must be determined, the camera must have good linearity correction, and the mechanical rotation must be precise. Many problems that have only a small effect on planar images can cause serious artifacts in SPECT imaging. For example, a slight misalignment of collimator holes typically produces loss of resolution or a circular ring artifact in SPECT images.

ITEMS 114–117: SINGLE-PHOTON EMISSION COMPUTED TOMOGRAPHIC ATTENUATION CORRECTION

Answers: 114, *T*; 115, *T*; 116, *T*; 117, *F*

Accurate imaging reconstruction in SPECT imaging requires data from full 360° data collection properly corrected for attenuation. In cardiac imaging it is usual to collect projection data in a 180° arc because attenuation severely reduces the quantity and reliability of the projection data collected from the right side of the body. Reducing the data collection arc to 180° is an expedient compromise because it also reduces data collection time by a factor of 2, but it causes some reduction in the accuracy of the reconstructed images.

Attenuation correction using a transmission scan is the most accurate method because the actual attenuation coefficients can be determined from the transmission scan. This is not done very frequently in SPECT imaging because the collection of transmission images usually doubles the patient scanning time.

Assuming tissue attenuation coefficients to be uniform can be justified in brain imaging or in body imaging below the lungs. In cardiac imaging the assumption of uniform tissue attenuation leads to some distortions in the data because lung tissue has much lower attenuation effects than muscle, fat, or bone.

REFERENCES

1. Hoffman EJ. 180 Degree compared with 360 degree sampling in SPECT. *J Nucl Med* 1982;23:745–747.
2. Knesaurek K, King MA, Glick SJ, et al. Investigation of causes of geometric distortion in 180° and 360° angular sampling. *J Nucl Med* 1989;30:1666.

ITEMS 118–121: IMAGE QUALITY DEGRADATION IN SPECT

Answers: 118, *T*; 119, *T*; 120, *F*; 121, *T*

When PMTs are operated in the presence of strong magnetic fields, the electrons spiral, and the output signal is altered. However, all scintillation camera manufacturers use mu metal shielding around the tubes to essentially eliminate the effect of the earth's magnetic field. Nevertheless, fringe fields from magnetic resonance imaging instruments that exceed 5 g (the earth's magnetic field is approximately 1 gauss) are known to produce distortions in Anger camera images.

Uncorrected center-of-rotation errors greater than $\frac{1}{2}$-pixel size produce significant losses of spatial resolution. In fact, errors of more than 2- to 3-pixel dimension can produce images whose anatomic landmarks are unrecognizable.

High-count flood correction can be used to correct for detector and collimator nonuniformities. Removal of artifacts produced by these nonuniformities improves image quality. Nonuniformities are primarily caused by nonlinearity (distortion).

REFERENCES

1. Bieszk JA. Performance changes of an Anger camera in magnetic fields up to 10 G. *J Nucl Med* 1986;27:1902–1907.
2. Graham LS. A rational quality assurance program for SPECT instrumentation. In: Freeman LM, Weissmann HS, eds. *Nuclear Medicine Annual 1989*. New York: Raven Press, 1989:81–108.
3. Saw CB, Clarke LP, Serafini AN. Influence of zoom factor on centre-of-rotation of the SPECT system and on the resolution of tomographic images. *Nucl Med Commun* 1987;8:3–12.

ITEMS 122–126: SPECT ARTIFACT

Answers: 122, *F*; 123, *F*; 124, *T*; 125, *T*; 126, *F*

Uncorrected center-of-rotation errors produce a loss of spatial resolution in SPECT images. The magnitude of the loss is directly related to the magnitude of the uncorrected error. Movement of the patient during a SPECT study produces an image of poor quality, but there is no characteristic pattern. The SPECT data sets should be checked for motion before reconstruction. This can be done by looking at a cine of the projection images or by studying the cinogram, or both.

Uncorrected nonuniformities in the detector or collimator produce ring artifacts on SPECT images. The rings are centered on the axis of rotation, not in the center of the camera's field-of-view. The magnitude of the ring is directly related to the location of the nonuniformity, its size, and its magnitude. Although ring artifacts are generally recognized as such by their characteristic appearance, as in the example shown in Figure 3, their visibility depends on the amplitude of the ring and the organ being imaged. Use of a specific filter, such as a Parzen filter, does not generate ring artifacts.

ITEMS 127–131: COMPUTER-OPERATING SYSTEMS

Answers: 127, *F*; 128, *T*; 129, *T*; 130, *F*; 131, *F*

The operating system is a collection of programs that forms a bridge between the user and the computer hardware and software and performs nuclear medicine data acquisition and analysis. The operating system cannot compute ejection fraction curves, but it can accept keyboard input from the user requesting that a program that does compute curves be executed. If the program needs input from the user, it is the operating system that handles the presentation of that request to the operator on a printed page or on the display screen. Likewise, the operating system takes the response of the operator and handles the transfer of that information back to the program.

The operating system also keeps a record of where things are stored on the hard disk and in memory and calls on programs to control specific pieces of the hardware. The operating system programs allow a nuclear medicine program to control ADCs for data collection. During the collection, the data digitized by the ADCs are temporarily stored in memory, then sent to a hard disk. When the user instructs a computer to analyze SPECT data, the operating system takes the request from the keyboard, translates it, and sends it to the program to perform the processing of the data set. All of the "behind-the-scenes" activities are performed by components of the operating system. Display of images is a function performed by specialized display programs that control the display system and use the facilities of the operating system but are not part of it.

REFERENCE

1. Pickens DR. The operating system. In: Erickson JJ, Rollo FD, eds. *Digital Nuclear Medicine.* Philadelphia: JB Lippincott, 1983:60–80.

ITEMS 132–136: PROCESSING OF TIME–ACTIVITY CURVES

Answers: 132, *T*; 133, *F*; 134, *F*; 135, *T*; 136, *F*

Any data acquisition operation is subject to fluctuations from random events in the data. A time–activity curve can exhibit significant superimposed noise due these effects. To obtain useful information from such a curve, it is often necessary to perform some type of postprocessing to reduce the effects of noise. A running-average filter takes several points around each point on a time–activity curve and replaces the value of this point by the average value of that set of points. The filter then processes the next point in the curve in the same way. The result is a reduction of random variations in the curve that are due to noise. Under some circumstances, curve fitting might be used as a way to eliminate random noise, but this technique is not the most desirable. Fitting an exponential to a time–activity curve is sensible only in the situation where the expected result follows an exponential function. Even then, random noise in the data can influence the fit. Deconvolution of the time-dependent input function for an organ with time–activity data from the aorta will remove the bolus shape from the time–activity curve by removing the spreading of the function. However, deconvolution is very sensitive to random noise in the data and is not used to remove random noise. A low-pass Fourier transform filter can be designed to limit the high-frequency components in the data. Because random noise appears most often as high-frequency information, such a filter should remove much of the noise from the curve and permit proper analysis. A high-pass filter would have the opposite effect. It would remove the low-frequency data that represent the information of interest and would retain primarily noise components.

REFERENCES

1. Gelfand MJ, Thomas SR, eds. *Effective Use of Computers in Nuclear Medicine.* New York: McGraw-Hill, 1988.
2. Jones JP. Clinical imaging studies. In: Erickson JJ, Rollo FD, eds. *Digital Nuclear Medicine.* Philadelphia: JB Lippincott, 1983:105–154.

ITEMS 137–141: ANALOG-TO-DIGITAL CONVERTORS

Answers: 137, *T*; 138, *F*; 139, *F*; 140, *T*; 141, *F*

Analog-to-digital converters are designed to permit analog camera data to be converted into digital form so that a nuclear medicine computer system can process them. The ADCs cannot operate on data mathematically, nor do they store data as images. Rather, they are the interface components between the camera and the computer system. During data acquisition it is often desirable to be able to reduce the field-of-view of a camera so that information not directly related to the organ of interest can be excluded. To do this, a zoom operation can be performed at the time that the image is collected. This is accomplished by increasing the gain of the amplifiers that are part of the ADC. The hardware zoom operation permanently changes the collected data to reflect the selected zoom parameter. It should be distinguished from magnification, which is a software function in which part of previously collected image is made to fill the display. Magnification is a reversible process because the original data are not changed.

A significant problem for any nuclear medicine computer system is that the ADCs are subject to drift and other instabilities that can occur over time. If proper calibration of the ADCs is not ensured by making ADC monitoring a routine part of quality assurance, the images collected with the system may contain data distortions.

REFERENCE

1. Erickson JJ, Pickens DR. Signal processing. In: Williams LE, ed. *Nuclear Medical Physics.* Boca Raton, FL: CRC Press, 1987:39–57.

ITEMS 142–146: SELECTING COMPUTER COMPONENTS FOR A SINGLE-PHOTON EMISSION COMPUTER TOMOGRAPHIC SYSTEM

Answers: 142, *F*; 143, *T*; 144, *T*; 145, *F*; 146, *F*

Minimum computer requirements for executing both SPECT and static imaging with no cardiac work are one or more hard disks and an array processor to perform the reconstruction for SPECT imaging. Unusually large amounts of memory are not required, nor is it necessary to have optical disk storage or electrocardiographic inputs. The SPECT reconstruction requires the use of an array processor to make reconstruction times reasonable. Also, operation of a modern nuclear medicine computer system with the type of software that is available today requires that the computer, no matter how modest in its capabilities, has adequate bulk storage in the form of hard disks. Optical disks are useful for archiving data but are not required, especially if one of the hard disks in the system is removable and is thus usable for archiving or if magnetic tape is available.

REFERENCES

1. Keyes JW, Jr. Instrumentation. In: Ell PJ, Holman BL, eds. *Computed Emission Tomography.* New York: Oxford University Press, 1982:243–262.
2. Croft BY. *Single-Photon Emission Computed Tomography.* Chicago: Year Book Medical Publishers, 1986.

ITEMS 147–150: ANALYSIS OF IMAGE DATA

Answers: 147, *F*; 148, *F*; 149, *T*; 150, *T*

Thresholding is a way of changing the display of an image so that only a range of counts is displayed on the screen. Thresholding does not alter the original data; it only changes what the user sees. Smoothing filters are used to reduce the random noise effects on an image, making it more viewable. However, smoothing also reduces the spatial resolution because the filter reduces the effects of variations in the image. Edges and noise components are smoothed, whereas more gentle changes in intensity are retained. Smoothing filters, such as a five-point smooth, are implemented in the spatial domain and can be applied relatively quickly. Filters implemented in the frequency domain are often more elaborate and can provide superior performance than filters applied in the spatial domain. However, these filters require that the images be transformed by the Fourier transform, processed with the filter, then inverse transformed to produce the filtered image. These transformation/inverse transformation steps utilize more time than is required for the application of smoothing filters in the spatial domain.

Temporal filters can improve the appearance of dynamic data sets by smoothing out variations between images caused by noise. Instead of filtering across the spatial dimensions of an individual image, the smoothing operation is across the temporal dimension of a dynamic data set. The result is a smoother time–activity curve from a selected ROI.

REFERENCES

1. Gelfand MJ, Thomas SR, eds. *Effective Use of Computers in Nuclear Medicine.* New York: McGraw-Hill, 1988.
2. Jones JP. Clinical imaging studies. In: Erickson JJ, Rollo FD, eds. *Digital Nuclear Medicine.* Philadelphia: JB Lippincott, 1983:105–154.

Index